THE Forever Diet COOKBOOK

Lea -
To great food
and amazing
health!! :)

CHRISTIN BUMMER

ISBN 978-1-7359602-3-4

 This book is for informational purposes only. It is not intended to serve as a substitute for professional medical advice. The authors specifically disclaim any and all liability arising directly or indirectly from the sue of any information contained in this book. A health-care professional should be consulted regarding your specific medical situation before adopting this or any other diet or lifestyle change.

www.theforeverdiet.org

Table of Contents

INTRODUCTION

The Forever Diet

When I first started out with a plant-based diet in 2011, I had no clue where to start. I was pretty clear on what NOT to eat, but I wasn't sure what TO eat. I began binge collecting as many vegan recipes as I could find. I quickly learned the difference between healthy vegan and junkfood vegan. There is a huge difference! For future reference, I generally consider 'healthy vegan' to be synonymous with whole food plant-based.

I eventually found some recipes that were actually healthy. Unfortunately, I wasn't an expert in the kitchen and most recipes felt time-consuming. I knew there must be a way to make healthy food taste good without spending all day at the grocery store or in the kitchen! I was seeing such good results from eating the right food that I went on a mission to find a way to make it work. It needed to be sustainable for the long haul.

Over the next several years I committed to creating food that was fresh and healthy, easy to prepare, and most importantly, delicious! Not every creation was a success, let me tell you! But over the years, I learned more and developed a knack for finding good combinations. I also learned that it's ok to streamline the effort by batch cooking, freezing the excess, and reinventing leftovers so no one really knows they're leftovers! In fact, it's crazy NOT to do these things!

The result of many years of trial and error, and lots of kitchen experimentation is what I am now proud to deliver as The Forever Diet Cookbook. It is a compilation of my most often used recipes. Many are suitable for entertaining, but the majority are for everyday life, where you probably spend most of your meals anyway! I think you'll find them relatively easy to prepare, especially after the first attempt, and I hope you enjoy them!

When I created The Forever Diet system, I knew that I had to make the food the easiest and most accessible part of the program. It's the foundation. Without getting the food right, nothing else matters. In the pages of this Cookbook you will find the groundwork upon which you can build your future.

Sustainable success comes not only from eating the right food, but also understanding why it is the right food and how to make it work in the real world. In the Forever Diet Coaching Programs we teach a foolproof system. We offer knowledge, strategies, and accountability, all of which are essential for long-term success.

The Green Light Cheat Sheet is a tool to help you understand which foods may work best for your body.

If you're not already enrolled,check out **www.TheForeverDiet.org** for more information and upcoming programs.

Let's get cooking!

♥ *Christin*

Green Light CHEAT SHEET

GREEN LIGHT FOODS
No Limits! The More the Merrier

All leafy greens: Spinach, bok choy, kale, collards, romaine. cabbage, etc

All vegetables: Bell peppers, red beets, tomatoes, carrots, broccoli, cauliflower, celery, zucchini eggplant, onions, mushrooms, etc

Starches: Potatoes, sweet potatoes, squashes, plantains etc

Legumes: Lentils (all colors), chickpeas, black beans, pinto beans, kidney beans, mung beans

Whole Grains: Brown rice, quinoa, oats, millet, amaranth, etc

Fruit: Apples, oranges, plantains, strawberries, raspberries, kiwi, blueberries, grapes, blackberries, melon, cherries, bananas, and more

Preparations: Raw, steamed, boiled, roasted, or air-fried are all perfectly fine!

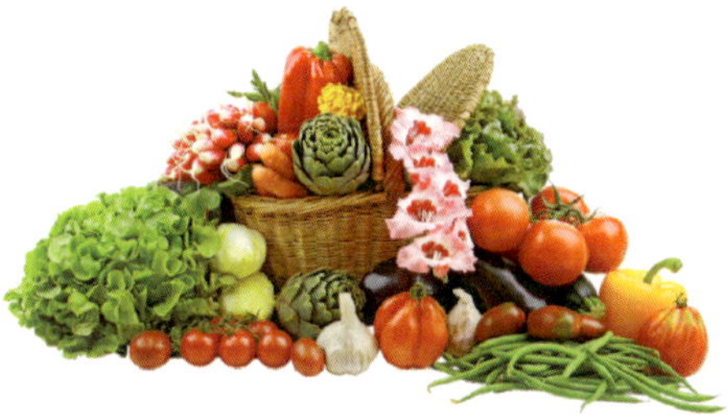

YELLOW LIGHT FOODS
Proceed with Caution. These foods are all calorically dense.

Nuts and Nut Butters

Coconut

Seeds (includes seed bread & crackers)

Avocado

Dried Fruit

Tofu, Tempeh

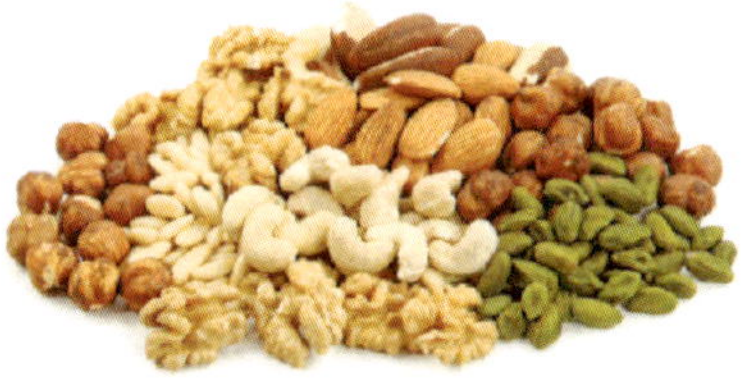

RED LIGHT FOODS:
These Foods Do Not Serve You! Stay Away!

All animal products: If it walks, flies, swims, or has a mother, let it be. That is, meat, fish, birds, eggs, or dairy.

All oils: coconut, olive, canola, vegetable, flax, grape, etc. This includes anything deep fried, cooked in oil, or with oil listed in the ingredients.

All highly processed foods: sugar, flour, alcohol, or products made with them.

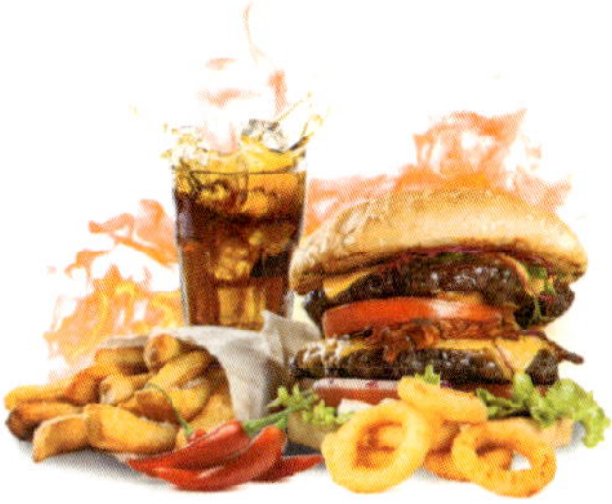

RECIPES

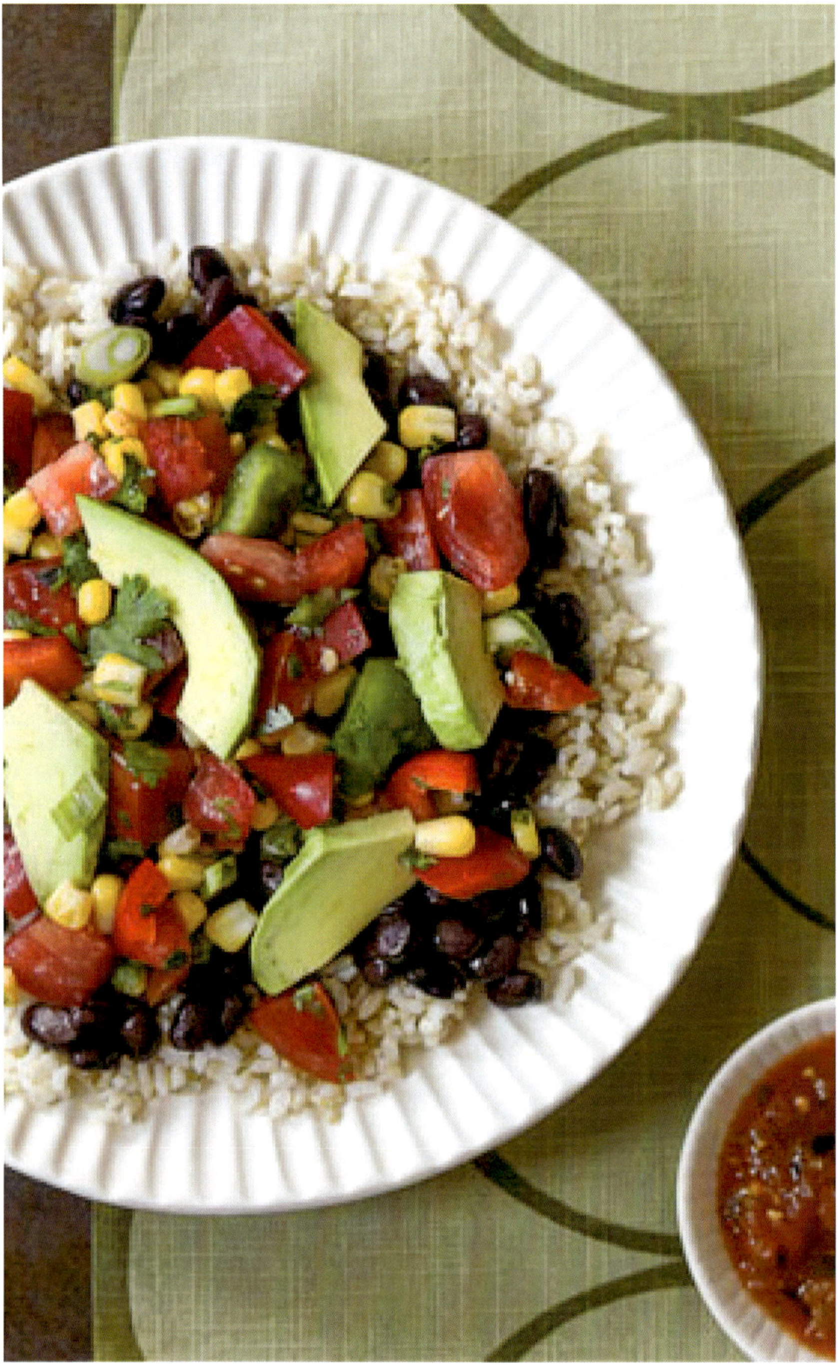

The Basics: Easy Food Fast

INSTANT POT VEGGIES AND STARCH

Sometimes we make cooking WAY harder than it needs to be. 75% of our meals in a week look something like this! It's nice to have the fun recipes, but it's also very freeing to keep it simple and realistic.

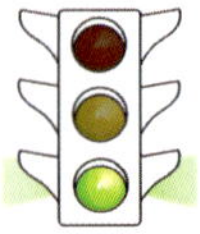

PREP TIME	COOK TIME	YIELD
1 Minute	Varies	Deliciousness

INGREDIENTS:

your favorite veggies

your favorite starches

INSTRUCTIONS:

Steam your favorite veggies, potatoes, and squash in the Instant Pot according to the following timetables. Your texture preferences may vary, but this is a general guide:

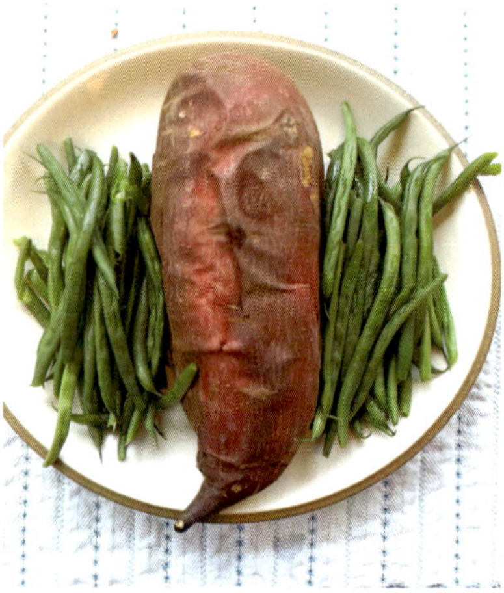

VEGGIES:

1 cup of water, QUICK release

Brussels Sprouts: 3 min (whole)

Green Beans: 1 min

Carrots: 1 minute

Broccoli: 0 minutes

Cauliflower: 0 minutes

STARCHES:

1 cup of water, steamer rack, natural release

Potatoes (cut into medium chunks): 4-5 minutes

Potatoes (whole): 8-12 minutes depending on size

Sweet Potatoes (whole): 10-15 minutes depending on size

Acorn squash, whole: 7-8 minutes

Butternut squash, whole: 25 minutes

Kabocha squash, whole: 8-10 minutes

Spaghetti squash, whole; 6-8 minutes

ZUCCHINI SAUTÉ

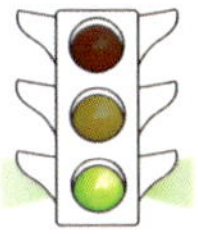

This is a great starter recipe for anyone who is learning to cook without oil. You'll be sautéeing without oil and I think you're going to love it! Master this one and you've got a great staple you can rely on. It's still one of my favorites!

PREP TIME	COOK TIME	YIELD
7 Minutes	10-15 Minutes	2 Servings

INGREDIENTS:

2 onions, diced

3 medium zucchini, diced

8 oz mushrooms, diced

1 teaspoon garlic powder

1 teaspoon onion powder

lemon juice or lemon balsamic vinegar

INSTRUCTIONS:

Cook onions over med-hi heat 2-3 minutes.

Add remaining ingredients and cook another 7-9 minutes to desired tenderness.

Add a squeeze of lemon juice or lemon balsamic vinegar.

Toss and serve.

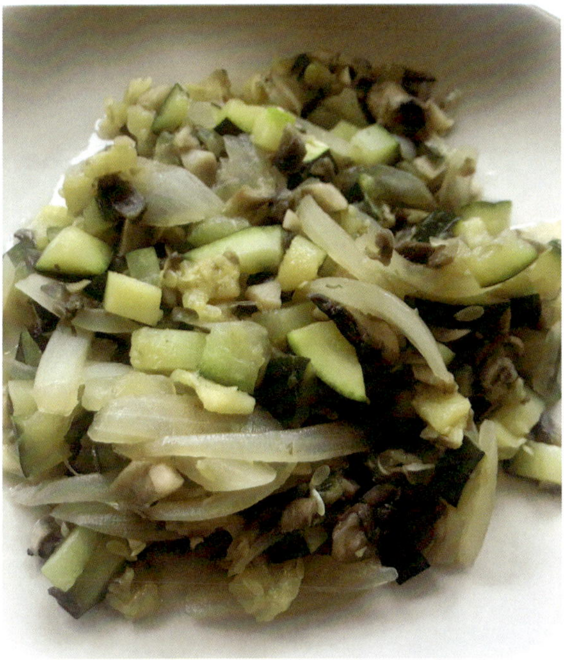

PERFECT AIR FRIES

I take great pride in my air fries. They have become such a staple and always fill me up. The coating for the Japanese Sweet Potatoes was perfected and contributed by my dear friend "Uncle" Jim.

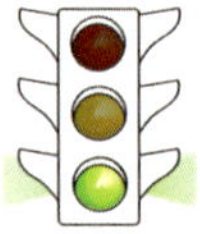

PREP TIME	COOK TIME	YIELD
5 Minutes	15-18 Minutes	2-4 Servings

INGREDIENTS:

2 lbs Yukon Gold potatoes

1/2 tablespoon garlic powder

1/2 tablespoon onion powder

OR

2 lbs japanese sweet potatoes

1/2 tablespoon cinnamon

2 tablespoons roasted flax seed, ground

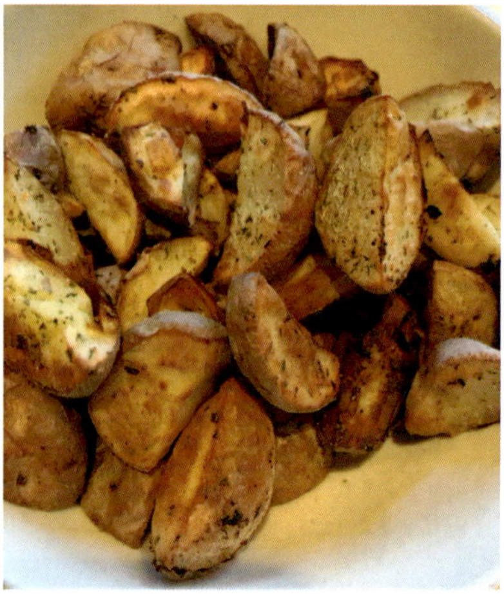

INSTRUCTIONS FOR YUKON GOLD:

Cut potatoes into wedges of roughly uniform size.

Sprinkle with garlic and onion powder.

Toss to coat evenly.

Cook in air fryer 390 degrees for 15-18 minutes.

Toss once or twice during cooking process and adjust time as desired.

Note: You can speed up the time and get a crispier result by using precooked potatoes. You can either roast a tray at a time in advance and use refrigerated potatoes. You can also microwave for a few minutes once you cut them.

PERFECT AIR FRIES CONTINUED

INSTRUCTIONS FOR JAPANESE SWEET POTATOES:

Cut potatoes as desired. I prefer thick slices, quartered, but you can do thin slices, cubes, or any other version that tickles your fancy. Experiment to see what you like.

Sprinkle a little bit of water over the cut potatoes for the coating to stick. In a separate bowl, mix the cinnamon and roasted flax.

Pour over the potatoes and toss to coat.

Cook in air fryer 390 degrees for 15-18 minutes. Toss once or twice during cooking process and adjust time as desired.

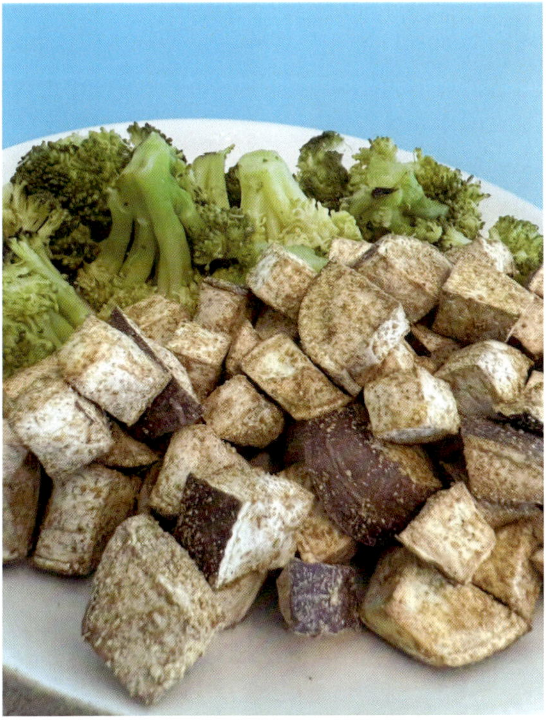

FIESTA FOREVER

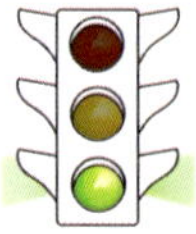

For some reason people have this notion that eating a plant-based diet is a life of deprivation, a sentence to living on "rabbit food." I beg to differ! If you're doing it right, it should feel like a party in your mouth, especially once your taste buds learn to adapt to the taste of whole natural food again. Once you arrive, it's a fiesta forever!

PREP TIME	COOK TIME	YIELD
10 Minute	15 Minutes	4-5 Servings

INGREDIENTS:

2 cups dry brown rice

1 onion, diced

1 bell pepper, diced

2 cans black beans
(no salt added)

1 cup frozen corn

16 oz salsa (salt-free is ideal but hard to find)

1-2 teaspoons Salt-free taco seasoning, to taste

juice of 1/2 lime

1 tomato, chopped

1 bunch cilantro, chopped

1 avocado, sliced (optional)

INSTRUCTIONS:

Get the water boiling for the rice first, or cook in the Instant Pot (4 cups brown rice with 5 cups water, 12 minutes at pressure plus natural release).

Saute onions and peppers for 5-7 minutes, adding water as needed to prevent sticking.

Rinse the black beans and corn and add to the saute pan with the veggies.

Add half of the salsa.

Bring to a simmer and add lime juice and 1-2 teaspoons saltfree taco seasoning at a time, as desired.

Simmer another 2-3 minutes for flavors to meld together.

Serve over brown rice and top with salsa, fresh tomato, and cilantro.

For a splurge, top with some fresh avocado.

Pictured on Page 6

STUFFED SWEET POTATO

This is one of those super simple concoctions that will delight your taste buds in a hurry. It takes minimal time to prepare, and is a great way to use those sweet potatoes that you've batch-cooked at the beginning of the week!

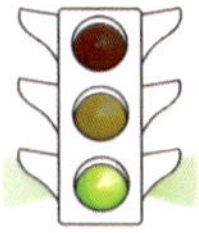

PREP TIME	COOK TIME	YIELD
2 Minutes	60 Minutes	4 Servings

INGREDIENTS:

4 medium orange sweet potatoes

cinnamon

16 oz crushed pineapple in juice, drained

INSTRUCTIONS:

Preheat oven to 350 degrees.

Arrange sweet potatoes on a non-stick silicone baking mat.

Roast for 60 minutes or until they begin to ooze liquid, whichever comes first.

Remove from oven and let cool 10 minutes.

Cut potatoes open (but not all the way through) lengthwise and squish the ends toward each other to open up the middle.

Top with crushed pineapple and a generous sprinkle of cinnamon.

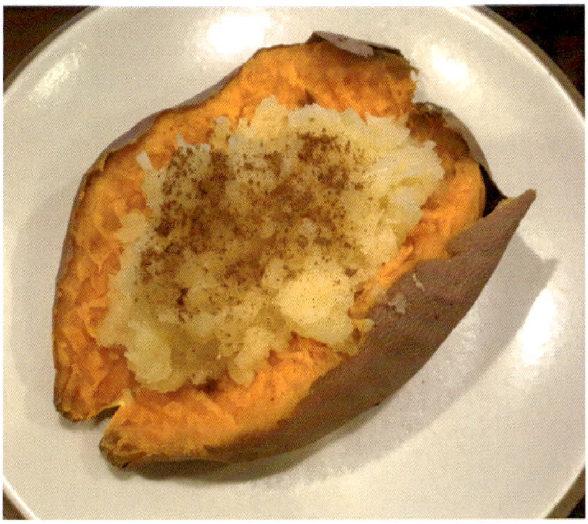

FRESH BERRY DESSERT

Try this simple dessert presentation next time you're looking for a healthy dessert that everyone will love. It doesn't get any easier or healthier than this. Mix it up with different berries, or just a different design. Garnish with fresh mint, and enjoy!

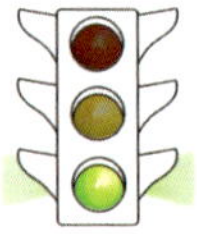

PREP TIME	COOK TIME	YIELD
7 Minutes	9-10 Minutes	4 Servings

INGREDIENTS:

32 oz strawberries

12 oz blackberries

fresh mint (optional)

dark chocolate balsamic vinegar (optional)

INSTRUCTIONS:

Wash berries.

Take tops off strawberries.

Layer on a serving platter in a pretty pattern.

Serve!

If you want to get really fancy you can serve in individual dessert glasses and drizzle with dark chocolate balsamic vinegar.

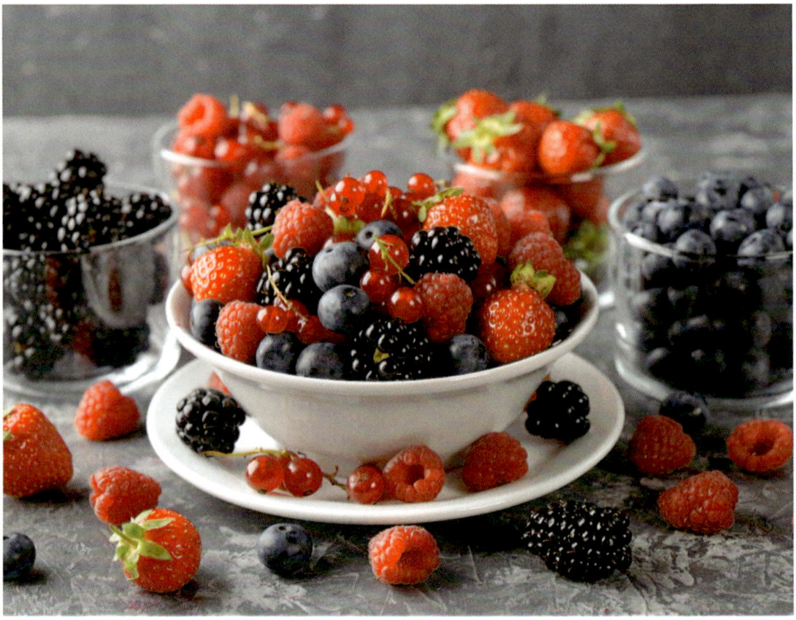

PERFECT JAPANESE SWEET POTATOES

This is perhaps the "recipe" that I talk the most about, and the one that gets the most questions. Japanese sweet potatoes are such a treat. It's important how to get the most out of them. Try these options as well as the other air fryer options to find your favorites.

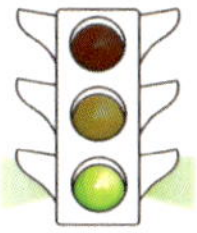

PREP TIME	COOK TIME	YIELD
2 Minutes	90 Minutes *(plus 12 minutes)*	4 Servings

INGREDIENTS:

japanese sweet potatoes

INSTRUCTIONS:

Preheat oven to 375 degrees.

Wash potatoes and arrange on baking tray with non-stick silicone baking mat. Do not prick skins!

Roast for 90 minutes and let cool in oven if possible.

Note - you can stop here and eat the wonderful ooey gooey Japanese Sweet Potatoes! You can refrigerate them, standing upright in an open container once cooled. You can eat them cold, you can reheat them, or you can proceed with the serving suggestions below for something a little fancier.

PERFECT POTATO SKINS:

Slice potatoes lengthwise and lay flat.

Cook in air fryer, face up, 400 degrees for 9-12 minutes. This creates a caramelized crunchy chewy layer on top that is reminiscent of the deep fried potato skins I used to love.

Check toward the end to make sure they're not getting too brown for your tastes.

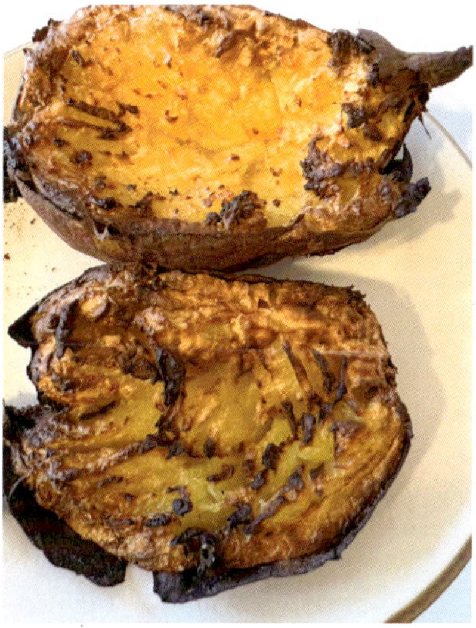

PERFECT JAPANESE SWEET POTATOES CONTINUED

HASSELBACK SWEET POTATOES:

Without cutting all the way through, slice the cooked potato as thinly as possible. I find it useful to nestle the potato between chopsticks, which prevents the knife from going all the way to the cutting board.

Place potato in air fryer and gently open the slices to allow heat down in between them as much as possible.

Cook at 400 degrees for 9-12 minutes to desired doneness.

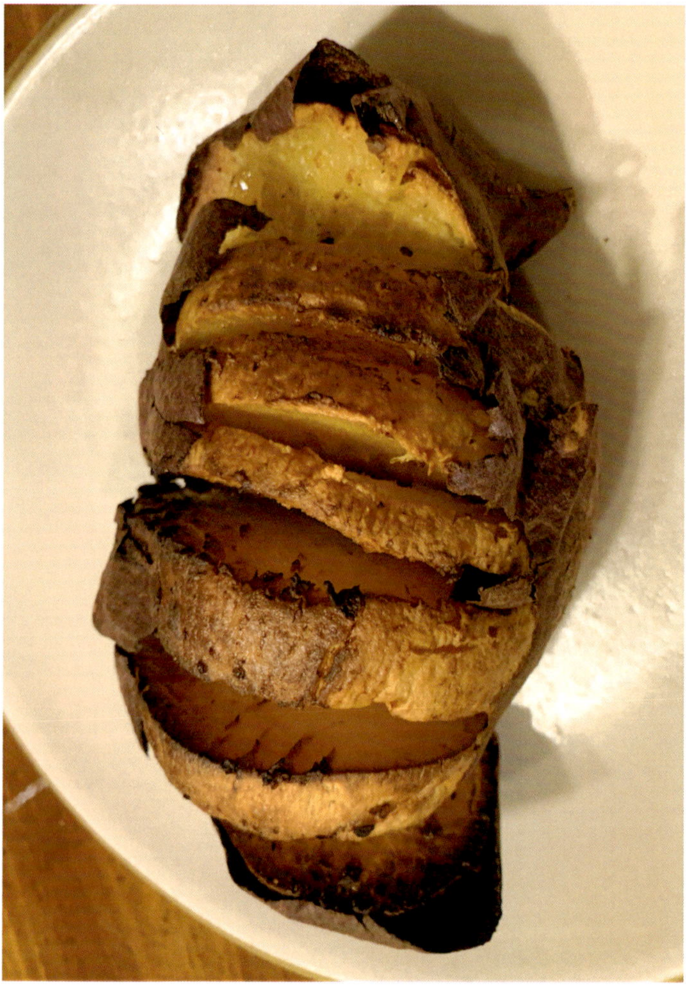

Rise and Shine

GUILT-FREE WAFFLES

This is my most-loved breakfast recipe. It turns a decadent splurge breakfast into something you can count as healthy and eat until you're totally stuffed without any guilt!

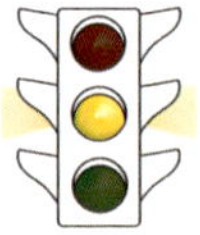

PREP TIME	COOK TIME	YIELD
5 Minute	20-25 Minutes	4 Classic Waffles

INGREDIENTS:

2 tablespoons ground flax seed

6 tablespoons warm water

2 ripe bananas, mashed

1/4 cup oat milk (soy and almond work great too)

1 1/2 cups fresh fruit, chopped. Raspberries, mango, strawberries, and blueberries make for a delightful treat but most fruit will work great.

1 teaspoon cinnamon

1/2 teaspoon vanilla

1 tablespoon chia seeds and hemp seeds (optional)

2 1/2-3 cups rolled oats

INSTRUCTIONS:

Preheat waffle iron.

Combine flax and water and set aside to thicken.

Combine bananas and milk first then add oats, cinnamon, vanilla, and optional seeds.

Stir in flax and water mixture which will act like an egg to bind ingredients better.

Spoon batter onto hot waffle iron, filling all the nooks and crannies.

Let run for the full cycle and then another 2-3 minutes.

Use a rubber spatula to peel the waffles off the iron.

Top with fresh fruit and a light sprinkle of cinnamon.

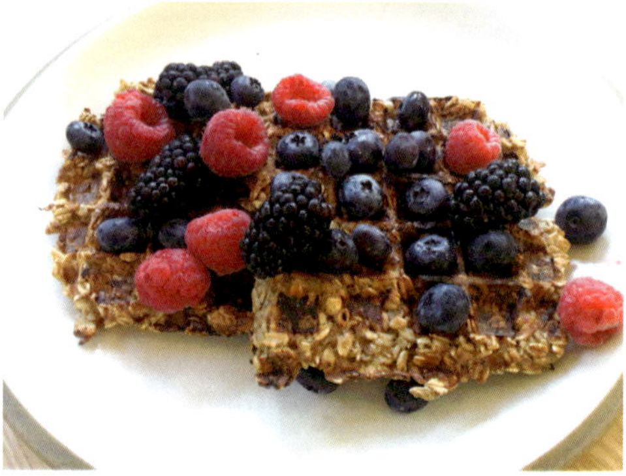

PUMPKIN OAT WAFFLES

This is a nice fall or winter treat when you just feel like something a little more pumpkin-y!

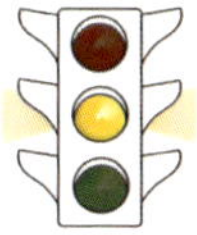

PREP TIME	COOK TIME	YIELD
5 Minutes	20-25 Minutes	4 Waffles

INGREDIENTS:

1 1/2 large bananas (or 2 small ones)

1/2 cup pure pumpkin (not pie filling)

1/4 cup almond milk

1/2 tablespoon vanilla

1 tablespoon cinnamon

1/2 tablespoon nutmeg

1/4 teaspoon allspice

1/8 teaspoon ground ginger

3 cups rolled oats

TOPPINGS SUGGESTIONS:

blueberries and raspberries

chopped mango

chopped pineapple

applesauce

diced apples and cinnamon, sauteed on the stovetop for 10 minutes while waffles are cooking

apple butter

pumpkin butter

INSTRUCTIONS:

Pre-heat waffle iron.

Mash together bananas and pumpkin in mixing bowl.

Stir in almond milk and vanilla.

Add spices and oats and stir thoroughly.

Spoon batter into pre-heated waffle iron, close lid and run for normal cycle.

When cycle is complete, lift lid to check for doneness.

All irons vary and your preference for texture will vary as well. On mine I like to heat about 2 minutes longer than the standard cycle so they're a bit firmer and have a little crunch on the outside when you cut into it.

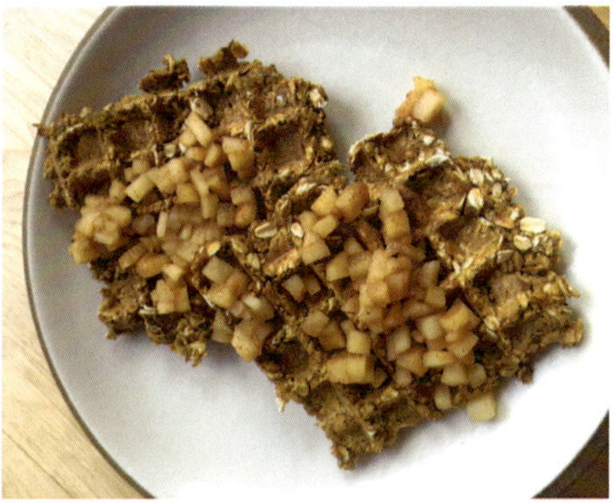

CHRISTIN'S POWER BREAKFAST

This is my favorite post-workout breakfast. It's packed with protein and heart healthy nutrients, with just enough sweetness to make it delicious.

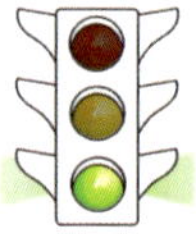

PREP TIME	COOK TIME	YIELD
8 Minutes	N/A	4 Servings

INGREDIENTS:

32 oz frozen chopped spinach

16 oz crushed pineapple in juice

3 cups cooked chickpeas (30 oz canned)

1/2 - 1 tablespoon cinnamon

INSTRUCTIONS:

Thaw spinach in colander under hot water.

Squeeze excess water.

Drain and rinse chickpeas.

Transfer to mixing bowl.

Add pineapple and cinnamon and stir with a fork.

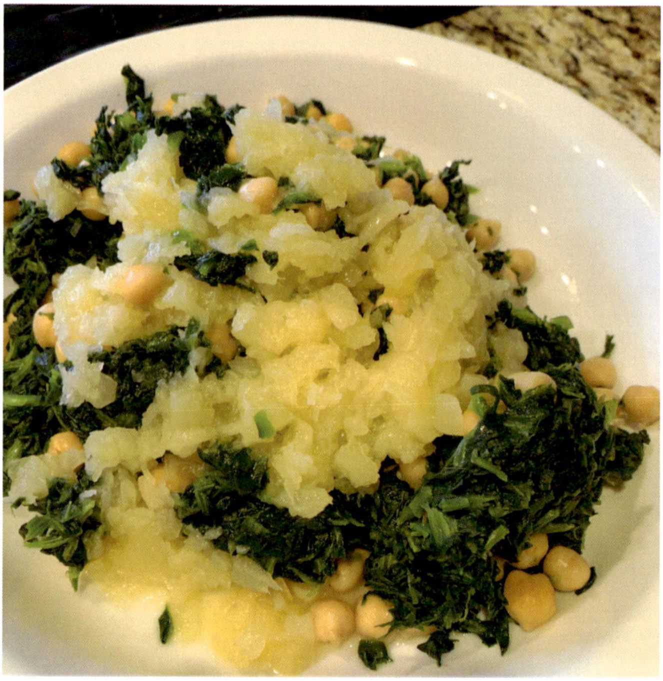

STEEL CUT OATMEAL-IN-AN-INSTANT (POT)

Steel cut oats were one of my favorite breakfasts for a long time. But they're so time consuming. It's so easy to walk away from the stove top and come back to a sticky mess. Not anymore! The Instant Pot take the guesswork out of it and you don't have to babysit it.

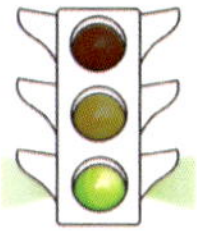

PREP TIME	COOK TIME	YIELD
3 Minutes	25 Minutes	6 Servings

INGREDIENTS:

2 cups steel cut oats

1 cup unsweetened vanilla almond milk

4 cups water

1/2 tablespoon cinnamon

1 teaspoon vanilla

1/2 cup dried apples

1/2 cup raisins

ground clove

INSTRUCTIONS:

Put all ingredients in the Instant Pot.

Cook on manual for 4 minutes. Let pressure release naturally (at least 12 minutes).

It may look too liquidly when you first take the lid off, but give it a good stir and by the time it cools enough to eat, it should be perfect!

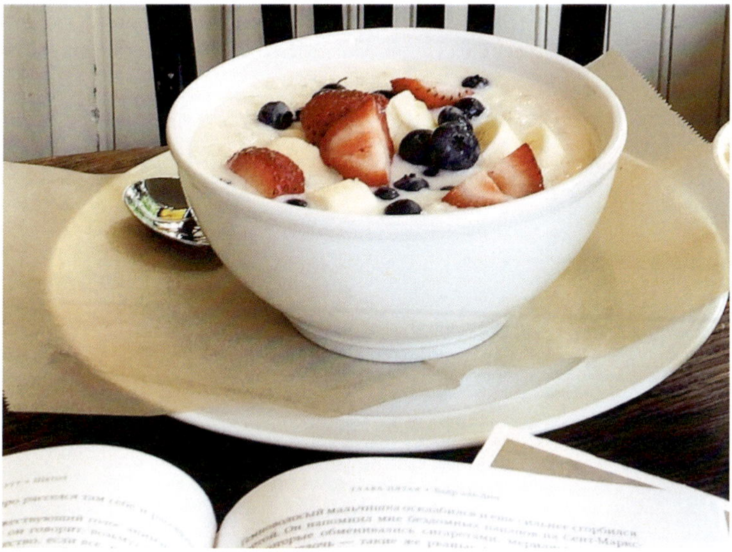

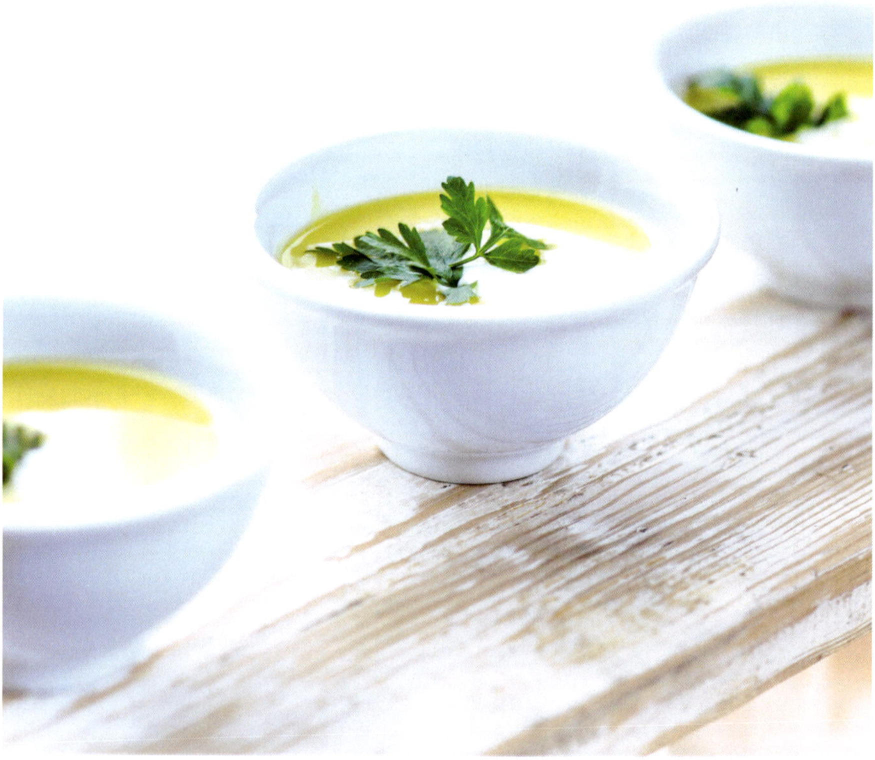

Soups and Salads

INSTANT POT BUTTERNUT SQUASH SOUP

If you're a newbie to cooking from scratch, this is going to wow your family! Just 3 ingredients, 4 if you count water, and you'll have a hearty soup on your table in less than half an hour.

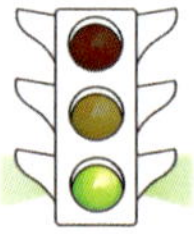

PREP TIME	COOK TIME	YIELD
3 Minutes	20 Minutes	4 Servings

INGREDIENTS:

1 large butternut squash

2-3 cups water

1 tablespoon cinnamon

1 teaspoon clove

Note – you can substitute almost any squash with this recipe. If you're not a fan of the spices, try omitting cinnamon and clove and simply use salt and pepper to taste instead.

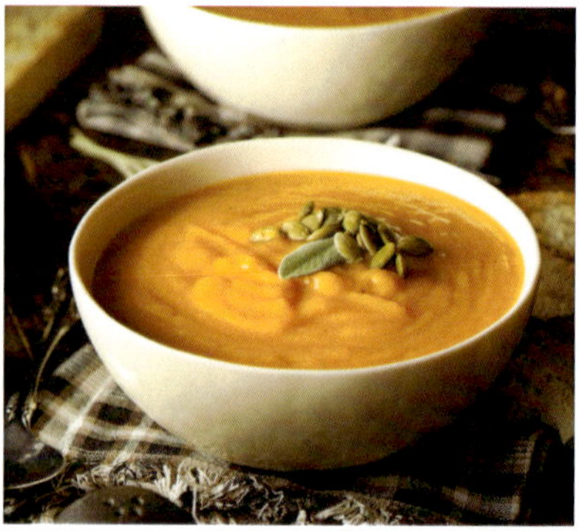

INSTRUCTIONS:

In an Instant Pot, place 1 cup of water at the bottom. Insert the steaming rack to hold the squash up out of the water.

Wash the squash and cut in half if needed to fit into the cooker.

Close lid, and set to cook for 4 minutes at pressure. (This will take about 10-12 minutes to heat up, then 4 minutes to cook).

When complete, release pressure slowly.

Remove squash, cut off the stem and the blossom end (the hard spot at the bottom).

Scoop out the seeds, but leave the rest of the skin intact.

Place into Vitamix with 1 1/2 -2 cups of water and spices.

Blend until smooth (~ 1–2 minutes).

Add more warm water to achieve desired consistency.

Pour into a cup or bowl and serve immediately.

A large squash will easily serve 4, if you're inclined to share.

SWEET AND SPICY KABOCHA SQUASH SOUP

When you're in the mood for a hearty warm soup that will fill you up without filling you out, you've got to try this! The squash is so satiating, and it's also great served over a bowl of brown rice.

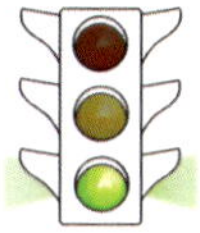

PREP TIME	COOK TIME	YIELD
10 Minutes	30 Minutes	8 Servings

INGREDIENTS:

1 kabocha squash,

roughly 2 – 2.5 lbs

1 cup water

1/4 teaspoon cinnamon

1 1/2 teaspoons Kirkland's salt-free seasoning

2 teaspoons Penzey's sweet curry powder

3/4 cup japanese sweet potato, roasted

3 cups water

1 1/2 cups unsweetened almond milk

2 teaspoons coconut extract

1/8 teaspoon cayenne powder

INSTRUCTIONS:

Wash the kabocha squash and place in Instant Pot whole, on top of the steamer rack.

Add 1 c water to the pressure cooker.

Place the lid on top, lock it, and cook for 7 mins.

When the cooking is complete, remove the squash carefully.

Let it cool until you can handle it safely.

Cut off any hard parts – the stem, the blossom scar on the bottom, any hard spots that look like barnacles.

Cut the squash in half and scoop out the seeds. Discard seeds.

Place the clean squash back in the Instant Pot, skin and all, with the steaming water still in there.

Add cinnamon, salt-free seasoning, Penzey's Sweet Curry powder, Japanese sweet potato, and 3 more cups of water.

Place the lid on top, lock it, and cook for another 3 minutes.

When the cooking is complete, remove the lid, and puree the mixture with an immersion blender.

Add almond milk, coconut extract, and cayenne and blend until smooth, adding more water or almond milk to desired consistency.

Serve alone or over a bowl of brown rice.

Pictured on Page 22

VEGGIE SOUP TEMPLATE

One of the tricks to cooking healthy meals in a hurry is being flexible and using what you have on hand. This is a life-saving veggie soup template that you can use to whip up a great veggie soup with whatever you have to work with!

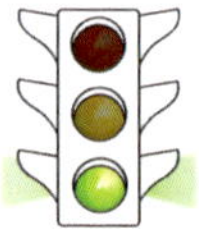

PREP TIME	COOK TIME	YIELD
10 Minutes	15 Minutes	6-8 Servings

INGREDIENTS:

4 cups veggies, chopped (think: onion, carrots, celery, zucchini, mushrooms, tomatoes)

1 cups starch (green or brown lentils, or white potatoes or sweet potatoes, cubed)

6 cups veggie broth or water

1 tablespoon oregano

1 tablespoon parsley

1 teaspoon garlic powder

1 teaspoon onion powder

1/4 teaspoon cayenne (optional)

INSTRUCTIONS:

Put all ingredients in an Instant Pot.

Cook on high pressure for 15 minutes, quick release or 12 minutes with natural pressure release.

Different combinations of veggies and starch will soak up the water differently, so feel free to adjust at the end by adding 2-4 cups more broth or water to desired consistency.

Variations:

Greek Lentil Soup - add extra 1 tablespoon oregano, 1/2 teaspoon cumin, 1/2 teaspoon coriander, juice of 1 lemon

Minestrone - a can of fire roasted tomatoes, spiralized summer squash for the "pasta", and a can of garbanzos

BLACK & RED PUMPKIN CHILI

Beautiful Black Beluga lentils are underutilized no more. They are packed full of nutrients including complete protein, vitamins, minerals, and loads of protein. They cook quickly and they hold their shape which gives a great texture to this chili. Adjust the spice by increasing or omitting the chipotle powder as desired.

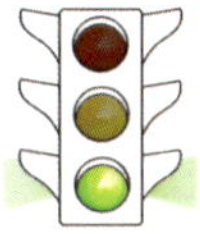

PREP TIME	COOK TIME	YIELD
12 Minutes	25 Minutes	8 Servings

INGREDIENTS:

2 medium onions, chopped

1 1/2 teaspoons garlic powder

1 teaspoon cumin

1 teaspoon oregano

1 teaspoon smoked paprika

1/4 teaspoon chipotle powder

Benson's Table Tasty

1 1/2 teaspoons balsamic vinegar

15 oz kidney beans, canned

1 cup black beluga lentils

1/4 cup red lentils

4-5 cups water

1 cup pumpkin purée

1/4 cup tomato paste

15 oz black beans, canned

1 lb corn

INSTRUCTIONS:

Using the Instant Pot on sauté function, cook onion until translucent, adding water as needed to prevent sticking.

Add dry spices and cook 1 more minute.

Add lentils, water, pumpkin, and tomato.

Cook another minute.

Close and seal lid and cook at high pressure for 10 minutes.

Allow pressure to release naturally for 10 minutes.

Remove cover, add remaining ingredients. Stir and serve.

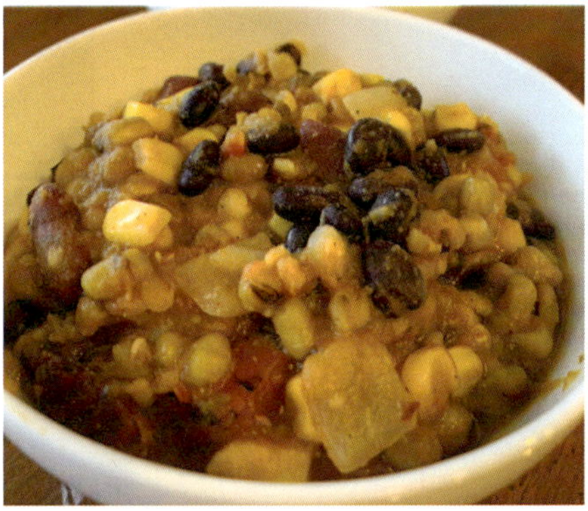

WELCOME HOME IN-AN-INSTANT (POT) CHILI

I love to travel and I often come home to an empty fridge. One time I went to the pantry and pulled out a bunch of ingredients and created this chili!

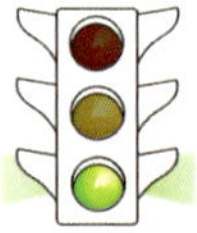

PREP TIME	COOK TIME	YIELD
20 Minutes	50 Minutes	8 Servings

INGREDIENTS:

3 15 oz cans diced tomatoes

2 15 oz cans kidney beans, drained and rinsed

1 15 oz can black beans, drained and rinsed

1 cup yellow split peas

1/2 cup red lentils

1/2 cup quinoa

1 large onion, chopped

2 cups water

2 medium japanese sweet potatoes, diced

1 1/2 tablespoons Kirkland's no-salt seasoning

1 teaspoon garlic powder

1/2 tablespoon onion powder

1/2 teaspoon chili powder

1/2 teaspoon cinnamon

1/4 teaspoon chipotle powder (optional)

INSTRUCTIONS:

Put all ingredients into an Instant Pot.

Cook on manual for 8 minutes.

Serve in a bowl or over rice, quinoa, or oat groats.

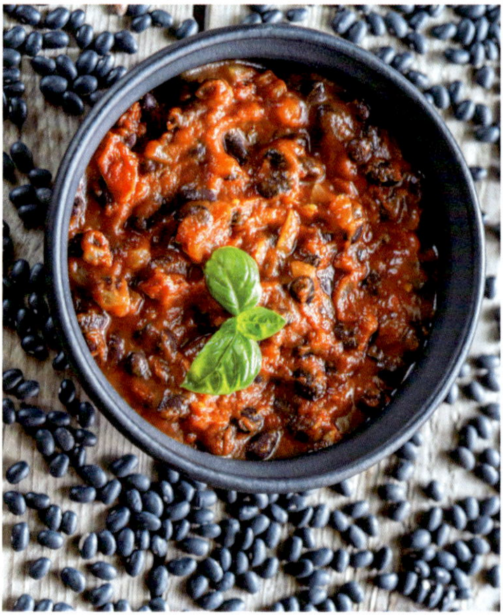

FRUIT SALAD

We're redefining fast food with this one! Here is a quick and easy fruit salad recipe. It's as colorful and delicious as it is healthy. Simply scale up as needed for a bigger crowd.

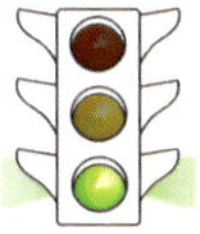

PREP TIME	COOK TIME	YIELD
5 Minutes	N/A	2 Servings

INGREDIENTS:

1 large green apple

2 kiwi

4 strawberries

1 tablespoon fresh lemon juice

walnut halves, optional

INSTRUCTIONS:

Cut all fruit into bite-sized pieces.

Put the fruit in a salad bowl, add the lemon juice to preserve color, and toss gently.

Add walnuts on top if using.

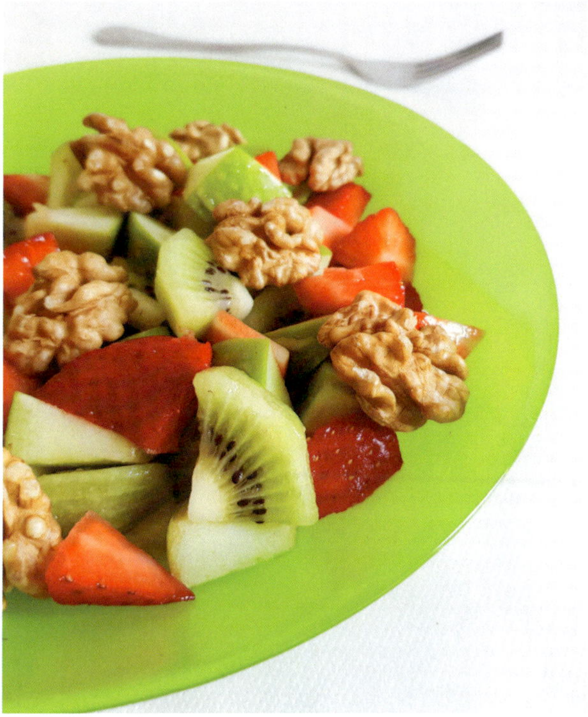

MOROCCAN SALAD

And now, for a staple that can be found on all Moroccan tables: a salad of tomatoes and cucumbers and warm spices. It's perfect to accompany your meal, or make extra and add chickpeas to make it a more filling meal.

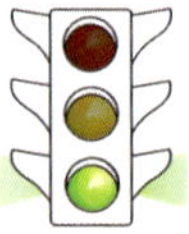

PREP TIME	COOK TIME	YIELD
5 Minutes	N/A	2-3 Servings

INGREDIENTS:

2 cups cherry tomatoes, sliced

1 cucumber, peeled and diced

2 tablespoons shallot, minced

2 tablespoons lemon juice

1/4 teaspoon ginger, ground

1/4 teaspoon cardamom

1/8 teaspoon cayenne

1/4 teaspoon allspice

1 pinch black pepper

red or green leaf lettuce

INSTRUCTIONS:

Put the tomatoes, cucumber and shallot in a bowl.

In a separate small bowl, combine the lemon juice and spices.

Whisk together until smooth and add to tomatoes and cucumbers.

Chill until ready to serve.

Serve as-is or on top of red or green leaf lettuce.

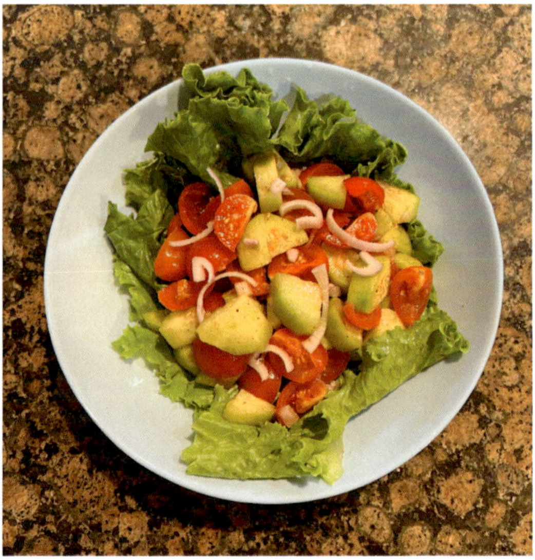

CHICKPEA SALAD

If I was stranded on a deserted island and could only take one food item with me, it would be chickpeas. Or maybe Japanese Sweet Potatoes. Or chickpeas... It's a toss-up. Either way, this fresh salad is composed of carrots, chickpeas, and avocado. It's tasty in all the right ways!

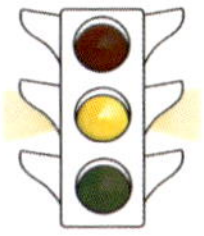

PREP TIME	COOK TIME	YIELD
5 Minutes	N/A	6 Servings

INGREDIENTS:

2 avocados, cubed

2 cups chickpeas, cooked or canned, rinsed and drained

2 carrots, grated
(or chopped if you prefer a crunch)

4 tablespoons lemon juice

1 teaspoon ground ginger

INSTRUCTIONS:

In a large bowl, combine lemon juice and ginger, mix well.

Add the chickpeas, avocados, and carrots.

Toss or stir gently until the ingredients are generously coated.

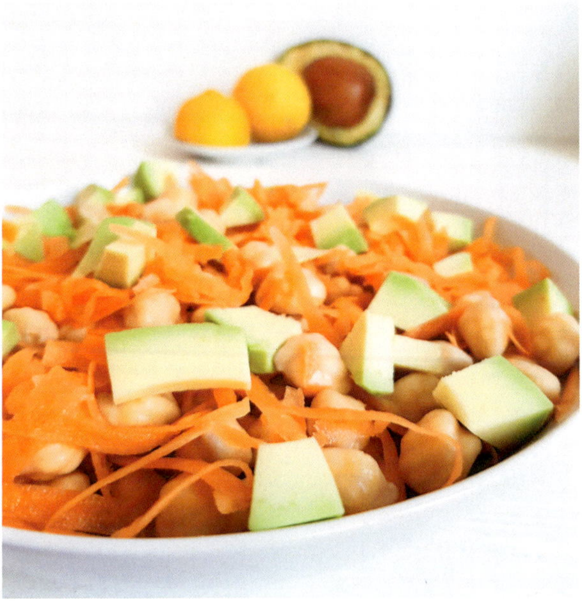

MANGO CUCUMBER QUINOA SALAD

Looking for a fresh and unique salad to take to a summer picnic? This is the one! Lots of fresh flavors without a ton of ingredients or prep time.

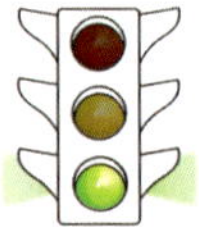

PREP TIME	COOK TIME	YIELD
10 Minutes	15 Minutes	10 Servings

INGREDIENTS:

5 cups cooked quinoa, cooled*

1 cup frozen corn, thawed

1 cup cucumber, sliced or chopped

1 cup cherry tomatoes, halved

1 cup mango, chopped

juice of 1 lime

1/3 cup lemon white balsamic vinegar

Note:

Quinoa:

Using an Instant Pot makes cooking quinoa (and everything!) a breeze. Be sure to always rinse quinoa thoroughly. Rather than the typical 2:1 ratio of water to grain, use only 1 3/4: 1. Set pressure cooker to manual for only 1 minute. Quick release.

Vinegar:

I order a few varieties of balsamic vinegar from www.theolivetap.com and californiabalsamic.com to keep on hand for precisely this purpose.

INSTRUCTIONS:

Cook quinoa according to directions (Instant Pot tips below).

Stir together quinoa, corn, cucumber, cherry tomatoes, and mango and set aside.

Combine lime juice and balsamic vinegar.

Pour over quinoa mixture and stir gently.

Serve immediately, or cover and refrigerate to enjoy later.

This is a super easy salad to prep ahead for summer BBQs or picnics. It's even better after being refrigerated overnight. If it seems dry, add a drizzle of balsamic and toss just before serving.

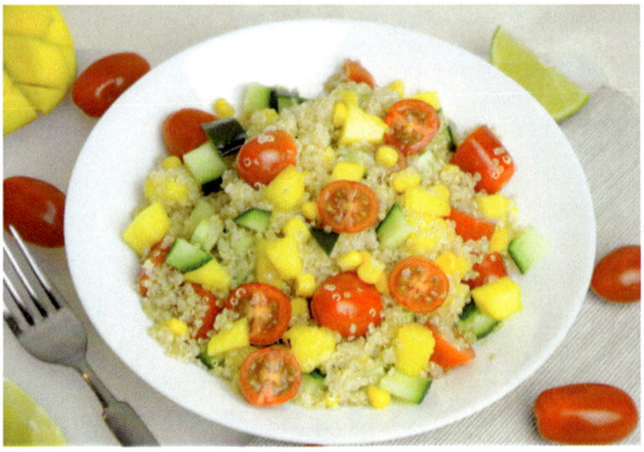

Main Dishes

VEGGIE STIR-FRY

There's nothing simpler than a Veggie Stir-Fry to enjoy the flavors of fresh veggies in a hurry! Swap out whatever veggies you prefer, try it with a different sauce, serve it over a different grain, and you can change it up every time you make it. Use this as a template to get you started.

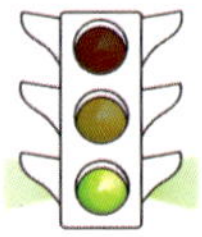

PREP TIME	COOK TIME	YIELD
10 Minutes	10 Minutes	4 Servings

INGREDIENTS:

4 cups brown rice, cooked

1 onion

1/2 lb asparagus

1 head broccoli

1 zucchini

2 red bell peppers

8 oz mushrooms

water chestnuts

bamboo shoots

IDEAL SAUCES:

terriyaki balsamic vinegar from California Balsamic

curry balsamic from California Balsamic

serrano pepper honey balsamic vinegar from The Olive Tap

coconut white riserva balsamic vinegar from The Olive Tap

ALTERNATE HOMEMADE SAUCE HIGH IN SODIUM, USE WITH CAUTION:

3 tablespoons low-sodium soy sauce

2 tablespoons lemon juice

1 clove garlic, minced

1/2 inch ginger root, minced

INSTRUCTIONS:

Start cooking rice in Instant Pot or on stove top.

Chop all veggies into bite sized pieces.

Put everything but the mushrooms in a frying pan with 2-3 tablespoons of vegetable broth. Any non-oil liquid works here – any vinegar, water, soy sauce, or even water.

Saute the veggies for 3-5 minutes.

Stir frequently and continue adding small amounts of liquid at a time to prevent sticking.

Add the mushrooms, water chestnuts, and bamboo shoots and saute for another 2-3 minutes.

VEGGIE STIR-FRY CONTINUED

For homemade sauce, add straight to the pan: 3 tablespoons soy sauce, 2 tablespoons lemon juice (fresh is best), 1 clove garlic pressed or minced, and 1/2 inch minced ginger root.

Simmer over low heat 3-5 more minutes until the veggies are done to your liking.

Serve over brown rice.

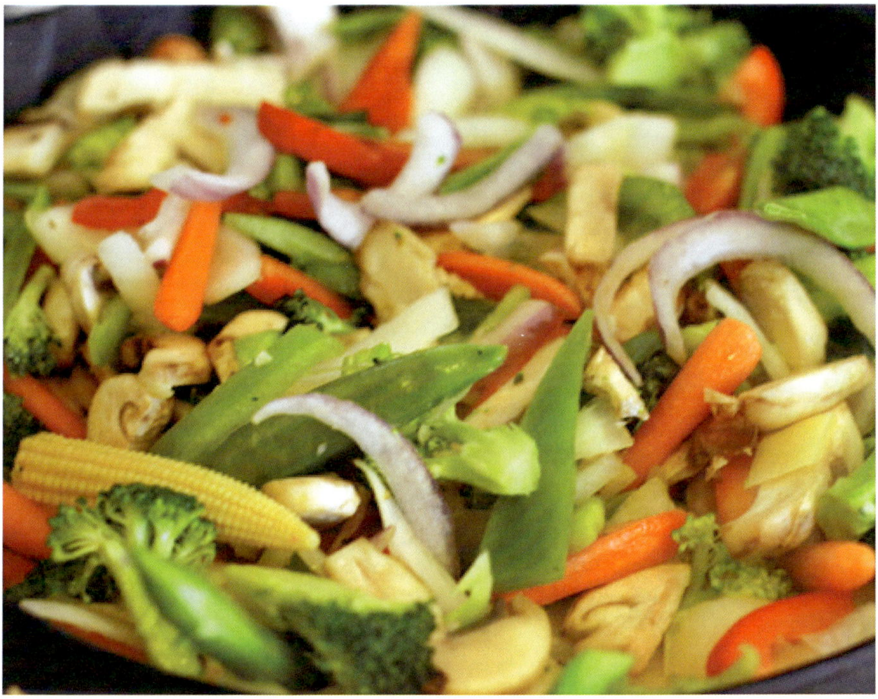

THE SKINNY ITALIAN SKILLET

Italian dishes are widely known for being rich in flavor and sky-high in calories. Cheese, processed meats, and olive oil are frequent offenders. But not here! Now you can enjoy all the flavors you love without all the guilt! This one is disease-fighting instead of disease-promoting.

PREP TIME	COOK TIME	YIELD
7 Minutes	9-10 Minutes	4 Servings

INGREDIENTS:

2 onions, sliced

2 cloves garlic, minced

2 zucchini, sliced

1 tablespoon fresh basil or

1 teaspoon dried basil

8 oz artichoke hearts, oil-free

8 oz cherry tomatoes

lemon juice

INSTRUCTIONS:

In a large skillet or wok, cook onions 3-4 minutes, adding 1-2 tablespoon water as needed to prevent sticking.

Add garlic and zucchini and cook 3-4 more minutes.

Add artichokes and cherry tomatoes and a squeeze of lemon.

Cook another 3 minutes.

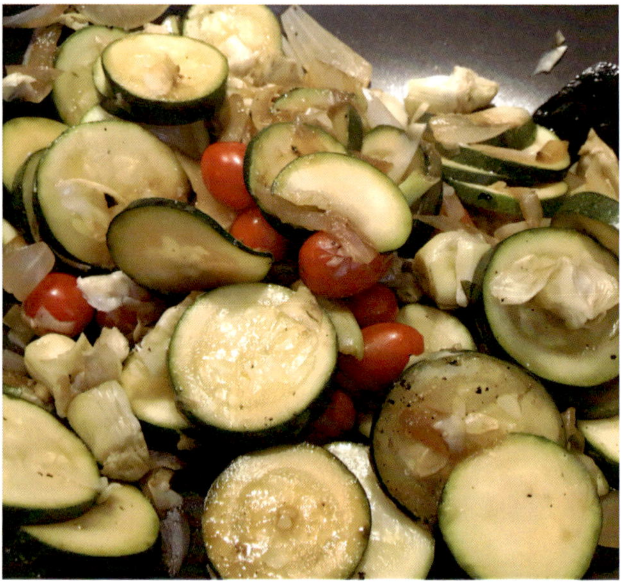

VEGGIE LOVER'S PIZZA POTATO

I once was at an Italian restaurant that had nothing but a salad on the menu that would have been compliant. But, they had baked potatoes and pizza toppings. And voila! The Pizza Potato was born.

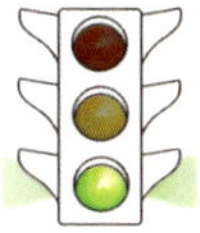

PREP TIME	COOK TIME	YIELD
10 Minutes	50 Minutes	3-4 Servings

INGREDIENTS:

4-6 yukon gold potatoes, baked

2 bell peppers, diced

2 red onions, diced

8 oz mushrooms, sliced

2 cups broccoli, chopped

1 teaspoon onion powder

1 teaspoon garlic powder

roasted red pepper hummus

2 cups marinara sauce

1/2 cup sundried tomatoes

pineapple (optional)

crushed red pepper

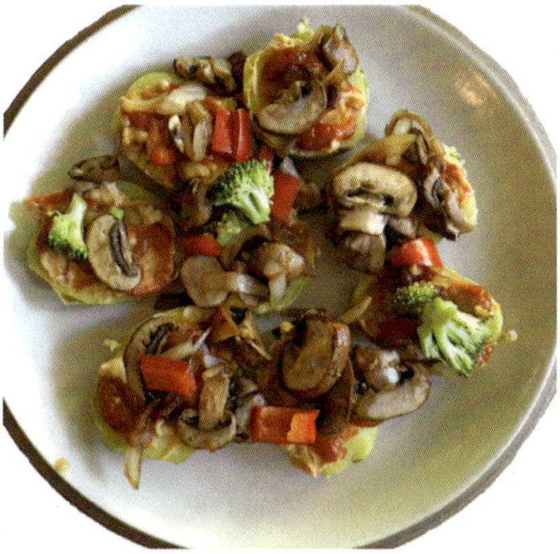

INSTRUCTIONS:

Preheat oven to 350 degrees.

Bake potatoes 375 degrees for 45-50 minutes.

Chop bell peppers, onions, mushrooms, and broccoli.

Sprinkle with garlic and onion powder, then roast in the same oven 20-25 minutes.

Split open potatoes, smash gently with a fork to form a flat surface.

Spread with hummus and marinara, then top with bell peppers, red onions, mushrooms, broccoli, and sun-dried tomatoes.

For more pizzaz, add pineapple, crushed red pepper, or whatever else you have on hand.

Return to oven for 5 minutes.

KHICHDI - INDIAN DETOX DISH

This is the traditional body cleansing food in Ayurveda and is becoming more popular as a detox dish in the US. Whether you're trying to detox or not, it's a delicious addition to any menu. It's simple enough to make regularly but tastes like a special treat. It's a comfort-food blend of soft rice and yellow split peas with just enough aromatic spices to delight your palate.

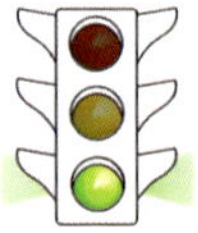

PREP TIME	COOK TIME	YIELD
10 Minutes	30 Minutes	4-6 Servings

INGREDIENTS:

1 lg onion, diced

1/2 teaspoon garlic

1/2 teaspoon turmeric

1/4 teaspoon cardamom

2 cups carrots, chopped

1/2 apple, chopped

3 cups brown basmati rice

1 1/2 cups yellow split peas

1/2 cups cherry tomatoes, halved

1/4 teaspoon ground ginger

5 1/2 cups water

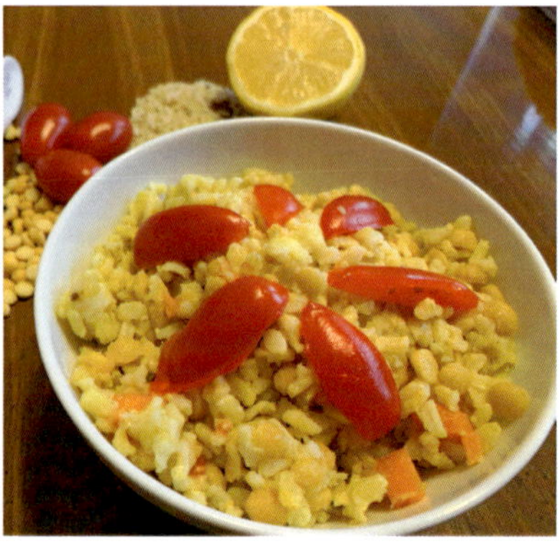

INSTRUCTIONS:

Saute onion in a few tablespoons of water in Instant Pot using saute function.

Add more water as needed and stir to prevent sticking.

Add spices and saute another 2-3 minutes.

Add carrots and apple, sautee 2-3 minutes.

Add rice, split peas and water.

Close and seal the lid. Cook on manual 14 minutes, then let pressure release naturally.

Add tomatoes and let sit another 5 minutes if possible (not mandatory!).

Note: Yellow split peas are completely different than green split peas! This is one substitution that would not come out nearly the same as the original dish.

SPANISH PAELLA

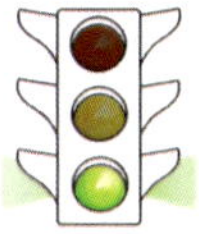

Paella is one of the most famous Spanish dishes. This vegan version is lighter and healthier than the traditional one, and is just as delicious! This is a little longer prep and cook time than most of the other recipes but it's well worth the wait! And the yield is really huge, so you won't have to cook for several days!

PREP TIME	COOK TIME	YIELD
10 Minutes	45 Minutes	6-8 Servings

INGREDIENTS:

2 onions, chopped

4 cloves garlic

1 red bell pepper, chopped

2 cups green beans, in 1 inch strips

3 carrots, chopped

3 tomatoes, grated

2 cups dry brown rice

3 cups water

1 pinch saffron

2 tablespoons paprika

1 tablespoon garlic powder

lemon juice

black pepper to taste

8-12 oz frozen artichokes, thawed

INSTRUCTIONS:

Instant Pot:

Put all ingredients into and Instant Pot. Cook for 20 minutes, then quick release.

Stovetop:

Saute onion in a large nonstick soup pot for 3-5 minutes.

Add water as needed to prevent sticking.

Stir in spices, potato, rice and lentils.

Add remaining ingredient.

Bring to a boil. Reduce heat, cover and simmer for 45-50 minutes, stirring occasionally.

Add extra water if needed to prevent sticking.

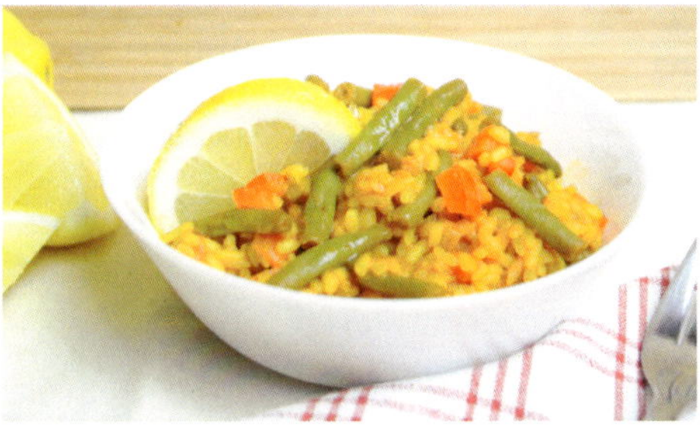

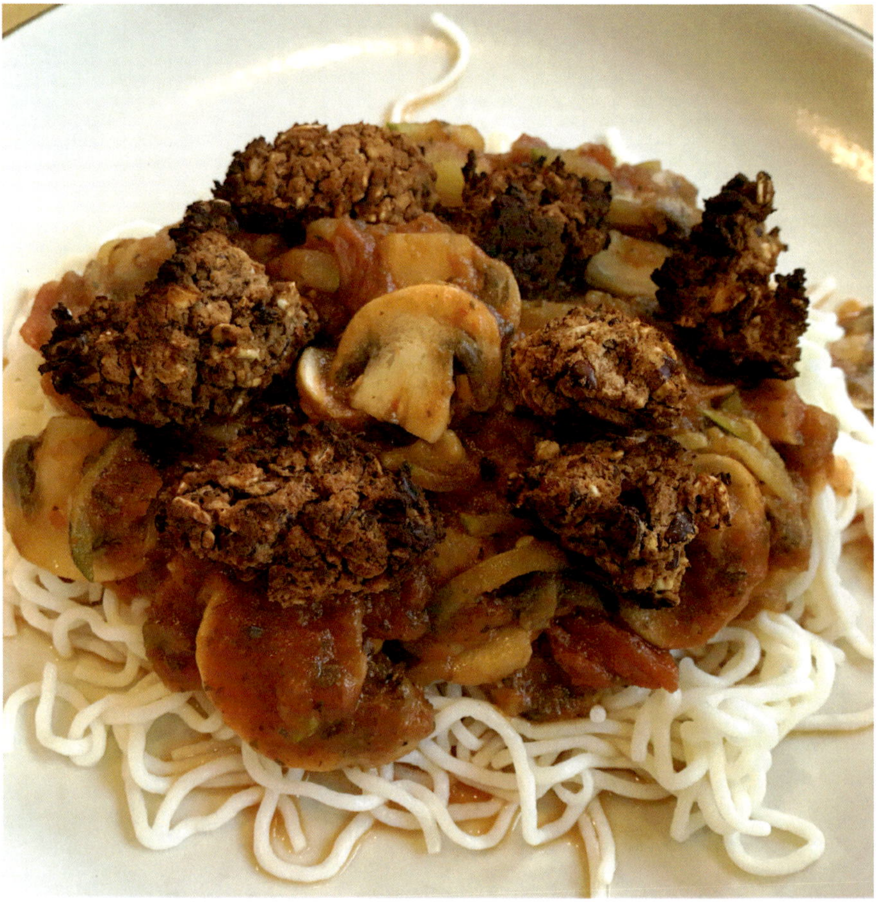

VEGGIE SPAGHETTI SAUCE

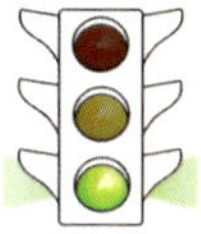

So many kids LOVE spaghetti and can't stand vegetables. This one should make everyone happy! It's packed with nutrients, but when you blend it at the end it makes for a nice consistency that should please even the pickiest of eaters. I love to serve this with homemade "meatballs" made from my Lentil Loaf recipe.

PREP TIME	COOK TIME	YIELD
10 Minutes	50 Minutes	3-4 Servings

INGREDIENTS:

2 onions

3 celery stalks

2 red bell peppers

1 zucchini

6 cloves garlic

2 cans fire-roasted diced tomatoes (salt-free if possible)

1 can diced tomatoes (salt-free if possible)

1/2 tablespoon basil

1/2 tablespoon oregano

1 teaspoon celery seed

1 tablespoon salt-free seasoning

1 cup water

1/2 cup red lentils

1 japanese sweet potato, roasted and cubed

2 tablespoons dried mushrooms

1/8 cup balsamic vinegar

1/4 cup white grape juice

INSTRUCTIONS:

In a large pot, saute onions, celery, peppers, zucchini, and garlic about 10 minutes, adding splashes of water as needed to prevent sticking.

Add tomatoes, spices, lentils, water, and mushrooms and cook about 15 minutes.

Lower heat to simmer.

Add Japanese sweet potato and blend with a stick blender to desired consistency.

Add balsamic vinegar and white grape juice to taste.

Simmer longer if desired or serve immediately.

Note: Serve over noodles of your choice. Whole food noodle options include Spaghetti Squash, Zucchini Noodles, Sweet Potato Noodles, and Kelp Noodles.
Other gluten-free options include Shirataki noodles, chickpea pasta, or black bean pasta and are great for kids or those who are not worried about weight-loss.

ZOODLES AND AMAZE-BALLS (OR AMAZE-BURGERS)

These "meatballs" were born out of a frustration with paying way too much money for frozen meat-free options full of oil and salt and mystery ingredients. Ick! They're AMAZINGLY easy, super delicious, and crazy versatile!

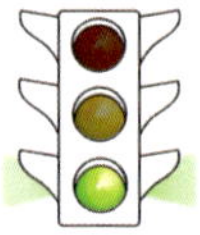

PREP TIME	COOK TIME	YIELD
5 Minutes	12 Minutes	20 Balls

AMAZE-BALLS INGREDIENTS:

2 cans black beans, rinsed and drained

1 teaspoon garlic powder

3 tablespoons tomato paste

3 tablespoons mustard

1/2 cup rolled oats

ZOODLES INGREDIENTS:

2 zucchini, spiraled

1/2 lime

AMAZE-BALLS INSTRUCTIONS:

Preheat oven unless using air fryer.

Combine all ingredients and mash with a potato masher. If you prefer to use a food processor, you can use that as well. Pulse until combined but not pureed.

Roll into balls about 1 tablespoon in size.

Air Fry for 12 minutes at 390 degrees or bake on a silicone baking mat for 18-20 minutes at 375 degrees.

ZOODLES INSTRUCTIONS:

Serve raw or lightly steamed.

Spritz with lime juice or your favorite sauce, and top with Amaze-Balls.

Variations:

Serve with marinara for a more **traditional spaghetti flavor**, or you can convert to a **hot dog style recipe** by adding 1/2 teaspoon liquid smoke or 1 tablespoon Hickory Balsamic Vinegar and form hot dog shapes before cooking. Serve in a romaine lettuce boat with ketchup and mustard.

If you prefer a burger patty, simply form patties instead of meatballs. I find these cook better in a skillet on the stovetop, but an air fryer works as well. Cook in a non-stick pan over medium heat for 10 minutes. Flip, and then cook 5 more minutes.

MEDITERRANEAN RICE

Move over South Beach Diet, this dish will run circles around you! Enjoy all the flavors of the Mediterranean Rice without all of the calories! The original recipe was formulated for the Instant Pot, but a stovetop version is shown below.

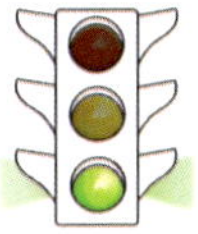

PREP TIME	COOK TIME	YIELD
10 Minutes	20 Minutes, then quick release	6-8 Servings

INGREDIENTS:

1 cup sweet onion, diced

2 cups sweet potato, diced

2 tablespoons Kirkland no-salt seasoning or Benson's Table Tasty

1 teaspoon garlic powder

1 teaspoon celery seed

1/2 teaspoon cinnamon

1 cup dried green or brown lentils

1 1/2 cups brown jasmine rice

1/2 cup sundried tomatoes, chopped

15 oz can fire roasted diced tomatoes

1/2 cup red or white quinoa

6 cups water

INSTRUCTIONS:

Instant Pot:

Put all ingredients into and Instant Pot. Cook for 20 minutes, then quick release.

Stovetop:

Saute onion in a large nonstick soup pot for 3-5 minutes.

Add water as needed to prevent sticking. Stir in spices, potato, rice and lentils.

Add remaining ingredient.

Bring to a boil. Reduce heat, cover and simmer for 45-50 minutes, stirring occasionally. Add extra water if needed to prevent sticking.

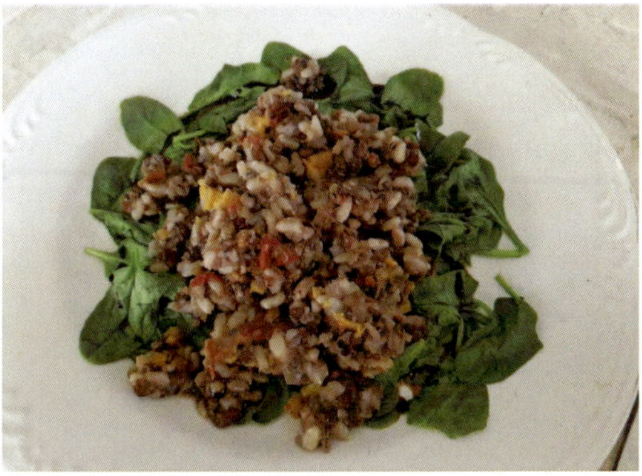

BURRITO BOWL

There's really no need for Chipotle when you can do this at home! I often use a base of brown rice and quinoa but you can certainly serve this over millet, oat groats or potatoes as well.

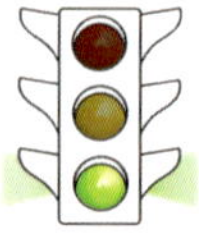

PREP TIME	COOK TIME	YIELD
20 Minutes	10 Minutes	3-4 Servings

INGREDIENTS:

Brown rice / quinoa blend

1 can black beans

1 onion, chopped

1 bell pepper, chopped

Salsa or fresh pico de gallo

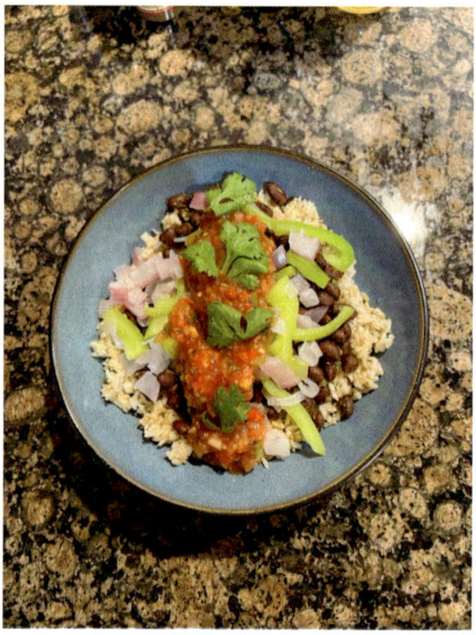

INSTRUCTIONS:

Prepare brown rice (in advance is ideal).

In the Instant Pot, add 3 cups of rice, 1 cup of quinoa, and 5 cups of water and cook for 15 minutes.

Release pressure and serve.

On the stovetop, prepare rice according to package directions.

Chop onions and pepper, heat in a non-stick skillet for 5-7 minutes, stirring frequently and adding water 1-2 tablespoons at a time to prevent sticking.

Heat black beans on the stovetop or in the microwave, optional. For me it's sufficient to drain and rinse under hot water.

Serve up your bowl with rice, then beans, veggies, and salsa on top.

Enjoy!

BAKED POTATO BAR

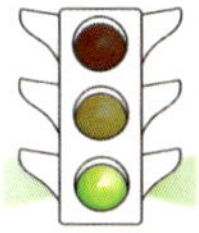

Pizza night or taco night has been transformed! This is always a crowd-pleaser and a great solution for families with mixed eating preferences. Each person can make their own variation. Kids can help chopping the veggie toppings, and decide what they want on their own.

PREP TIME	COOK TIME	YIELD
10 Minutes	80 Minutes	1 potato per person

INGREDIENTS:

Russet Potatoes or Yukon gold, baked

3 variations to get you started...

1. Taco night: Taco seasoning, lettuce, tomatoes, olives, and salsa
2. Pizza night: Spread with tomato paste and hummus then top with roasted peppers, onions, mushrooms, and broccoli
3. Broccoli and Cheeze Sauce (page 54)

INSTRUCTIONS:

Wash, prick with a fork, and roast whole potatoes (in advance is ideal) at 375 degrees for 50-70 minutes depending on size.

OR, you can microwave for 6-9 minutes depending on size.

Either way, turn once halfway through and cook until fork tender.

Add toppings and serve!

I like to make pizza potatoes the same time I'm roasting a whole tray of potatoes for the week, and I roast the pizza toppings on another tray for about 20 minutes as the potatoes are finishing up.

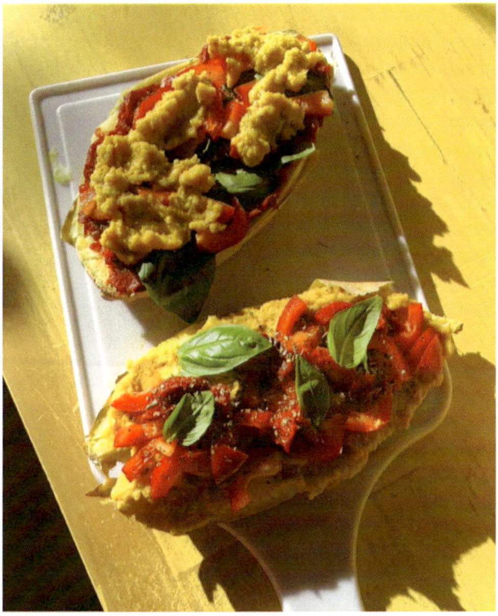

STUFFED MUSHROOM CAPS

This is my go-to entertaining recipe for special occasions. It feels like a gourmet restaurant meal but it's ready in a jiffy and has only 4 ingredients!

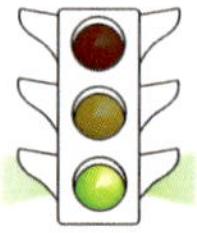

PREP TIME	COOK TIME	YIELD
10 Minutes	30-35 Minutes	4 Servings

INGREDIENTS:

3 lbs japanese sweet potatoes

1 - 2 cups unsweetened almond milk

4-5 portobello mushrooms (or 10-12 baby bellas, or white button mushroom caps)

balsamic vinegar

FILLING INSTRUCTIONS:

Chunk and boil potatoes (skins on if organic) for 10 minutes until they split easily when tested with a fork.

Drain. Mash by hand or with an electric mixer on low (do not use immersion blender).

Add almond milk 1/2 cup at a time until desired consistency

MUSHROOM INSTRUCTIONS:

Preheat oven to 375 degrees.

Remove stems and gills to clean mushrooms.

Place gills side up on baking sheet.

Drizzle with balsamic vinegar. Roast for 7-10 minutes for full portobello caps (less for baby bellas or white buttons).

Remove from oven and fill caps with mashed potatoes.

Roast for another 10-12 minutes until potatoes begin to brown.

Drizzle with balsamic vinegar to serve, if desired.

Note: These work great in an air fryer too!

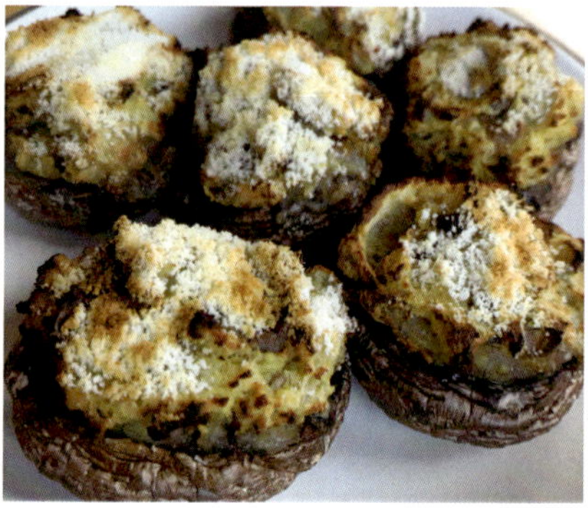

SWEET POTATO FALAFEL

I love the crunch and flavor of a good ol' fashioned falafel. But I'll pass on the deep-fried version, thank you very much! This version offers the taste and mouthfeel without all of the detrimental effects of oil. The slider-sized servings make for a fun finger food for kids too.

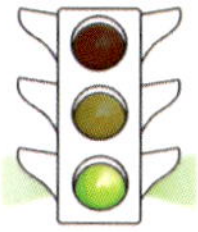

PREP TIME	COOK TIME	YIELD
5 Minutes	25-30 Minutes	4-5 Servings

INGREDIENTS:

2 cups chickpeas

2 medium sweet potatoes, roasted and peeled

1/2 cup rolled oats

1/4 cup dried parsley

1/4 teaspoon garlic powder

1/4 teaspoon cumin

2 teaspoons Benson's Table Tasty

INSTRUCTIONS:

Preheat oven to 400 degrees.

Put all ingredients in a food processor.

Process until mixture clumps together but be sure to maintain some chunky texture so it's not as smooth as hummus. Scrape sides a few times.

Roll into 1 - 1 1/2 tablespoon balls and place on silicone baking mat or parchment paper.

Flatten gently with the back of a wooden spoon. Bake 15-20 minutes until edges are browned.

Flip gently and bake another 10 minutes.

Serve with Harvest Hummus.

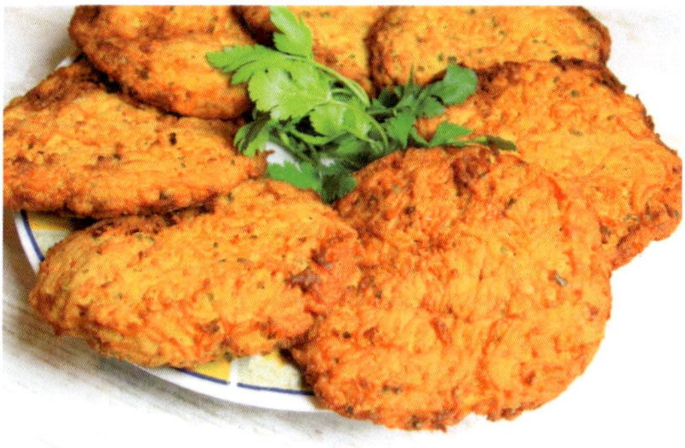

NOT YO MAMA'S LENTIL LOAF

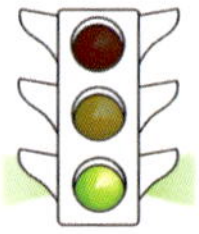

Having a good lentil loaf in your arsenal is a must for any plant-based household! This is such a great combination of flavors that it bears little resemblance to traditional meatloaf, by design... It is such a great way to get power-packed lentils into your diet on a regular basis. It makes more than a full loaf, so I love to make the extras into falafel-sized sliders. You can also double the recipe and make a week's worth of veggie burgers and freeze them.

PREP TIME	COOK TIME	YIELD
7 Minutes	80 Minutes	1 loaf plus extra for sliders

INGREDIENTS:

2 cups chickpeas

2 medium sweet potatoes, roasted and peeled

1/2 cup rolled oats

1/4 cup dried parsley

1/4 teaspoon garlic powder

1/4 teaspoon cumin

2 teaspoons Benson's Table Tasty

INSTRUCTIONS:

Pre-heat oven to 350 degrees.

Bring 6 cups of water to a boil.

Add lentils, cover, and boil 15-20 minutes until cooked through.

In the meantime, saute onions, carrots, and garlic 2-3 minutes.

Add spices and cook another 2-3 minutes, adding water as necessary to prevent sticking.

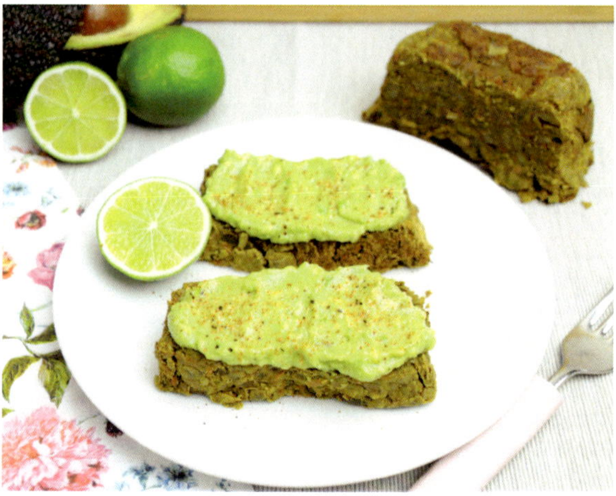

LENTILS AND CARAMELIZED ONIONS

This was inspired from a visit to one of our favorite Middle Eastern restaurants. Unfortunately, the restaurant version was laden with fried onions, olive oil, and gobs of salt. This one is just full of nutrition and flavor!

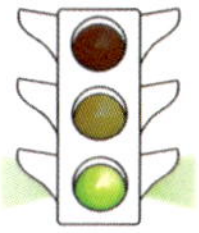

PREP TIME	COOK TIME	YIELD
3 Minutes	25-35 Minutes	6 Servings

INGREDIENTS:

2 cups dried lentils, brown or green

2 cups cooked brown rice

1 bay leaf

2 onions, thinly sliced

1 teaspoon cumin

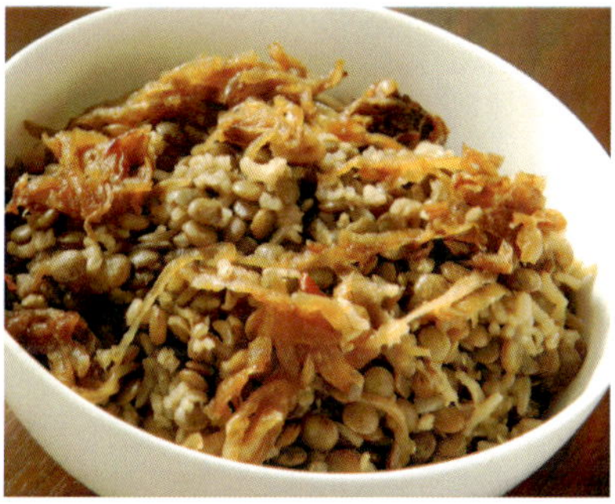

INSTRUCTIONS:

Lentils:

Follow package directions to boil lentils with bay leaf – usually takes about 20-25 minutes on the stovetop. Or 10 minutes in the Instant Pot.

Prep onions while lentils are cooking.

Onions:

Peel and slice the onions very thinly.

Keep in rings or cut smaller if desired.

Cook 5-10 minutes on med-hi heat in wide bottom fry pan.

Use just enough water or veggie broth to prevent from sticking.

Onions have their own water and sugar so you don't need to add much.

Once caramelized nicely, lower heat to simmer, stir in lentils and cumin.

Let simmer 5-10 minutes and serve over brown rice or all by itself.

A dollop of hummus on top can be a nice addition!

GREEN BEANS & KABOCHA SQUASH

This dish just screams fall. There is something magical about the combination of green beans and squash. The bright healthful colors look gorgeous together, and a drizzle of a nicely reduced balsamic vinegar turns this two ingredient dish into a crowd pleaser. Sometimes the simple taste is exactly what you need!

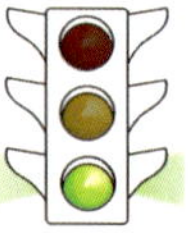

PREP TIME	COOK TIME	YIELD
3 Minutes	20 Minutes	4 Servings

INGREDIENTS:

2 lb green beans

1 large kabocha squash

balsamic vinegar

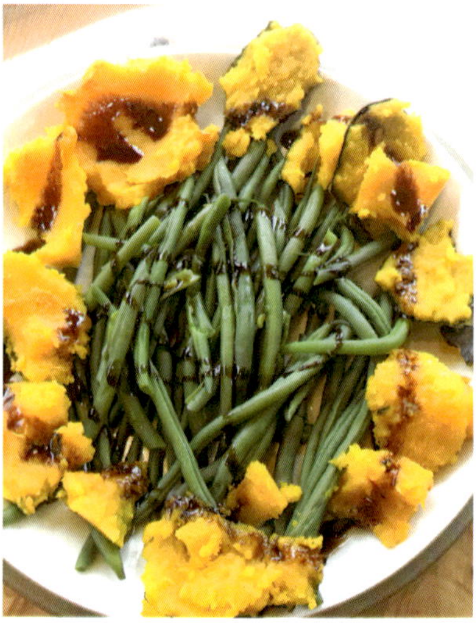

INSTRUCTIONS:

Put the whole kabocha on a steamer rack in the Instant Pot and cook for 7 minutes with 1 cup of water.

Quick release pressure.

While the squash is cooking, cook the beans in a large pot on the stovetop with cup of water.

Bring to a boil, lower heat to medium, cover and steam for 5-7 minutes to desired consistency.

When kabocha is complete, carefully remove from Instant Pot.

Cut in half and remove seeds and pulp.

Remove any bumps or scars on the squash's skin.

Leaving the rest of the skin intact, cut the squash into bite sized chunks.

Drain the green beans.

Cut into bite sized pieces if desired or serve whole.

Serve with squash on top and drizzle with a reduced balsamic vinegar such as Napa Valley Naturals Grand Reserve.

Hummus and Sauces

HARVEST HUMMUS

Try this delicious combination of power packed chickpeas and creamy sweet potato. With a sprinkle of pumpkin spice it tastes just like a fall harvest!

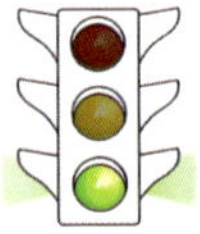

PREP TIME	COOK TIME	YIELD
5 Minutes	N/A	About 2 1/2 cups

INGREDIENTS:

15 oz can chickpeas

1 1/2 cups roasted sweet potato

1 tablespoon fresh lemon juice

1/2 tablespoon pumpkin spice

INSTRUCTIONS:

Put all ingredients in a food processor.

Combine until blended, adding 1/2 cup to 3/4 cup water to achieve desired consistency.

Serve with veggies, sliced apples, crackers, on top of steamed veggies, or add some water or broth to make a nice salad dressing.

Shown here with Sweet Potato Falafel. Enjoy!

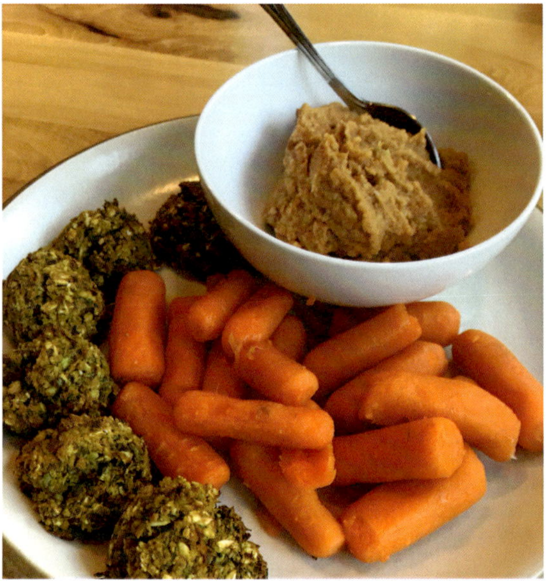

SWEET POTATO WHITE BEAN HUMMUS

This little twist on white bean hummus makes such a creamy delight, you won't even miss the oil. And, you can add all the protein and flavor you like without worrying about the calories of store-bought hummus.

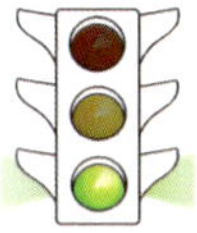

PREP TIME	COOK TIME	YIELD
5 Minutes	N/A	About 2 1/2 cups

INGREDIENTS:

1 large sweet potato, roasted and peeled

1 can cannellini beans, drained

juice of 1 lemon

1 clove garlic

1/2 teaspoon cumin powder

1 tablespoon dried parsley

INSTRUCTIONS:

Place all ingredients in a food processor and blend until smooth.

Serve with fresh-cut veggies or Sweet Potato Falafel.

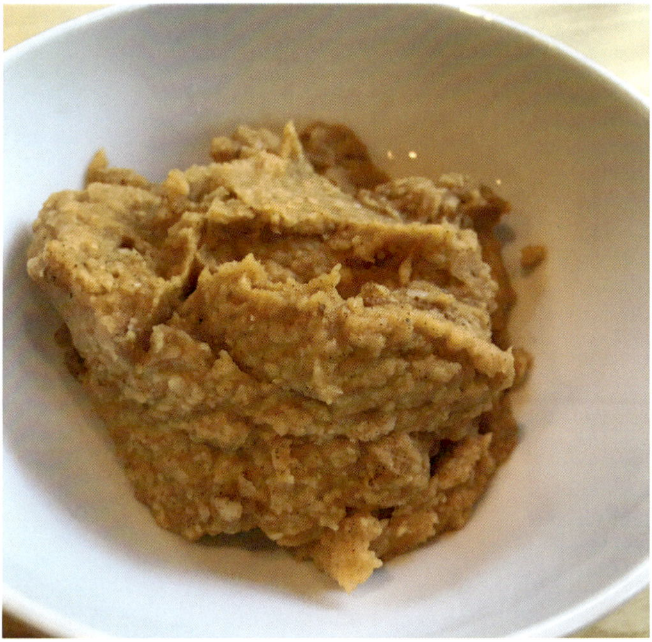

CHEEZE SAUCE

This sauce is great for the Baked Potato Bar on page 49!

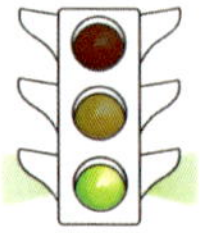

PREP TIME	COOK TIME	YIELD
5 Minutes	10 Minutes	20 oz

INGREDIENTS:

2 cups white potato, cubed

1 1/2 cups carrots, sliced

1 tablespoon onion powder

1 teaspoon garlic powder

2 tablespoons nutritional yeast

1 teaspoon lemon juice

1 teaspoon Smoked Hickory Balsamic Vinegar

INSTRUCTIONS:

Boil potatoes and carrots until tender. (about 8-10 minutes).

Reserve water from draining.

Add potatoes and carrots to blender or food processor with remaining ingredients.

Blend to desired consistency, adding cooking water as needed.

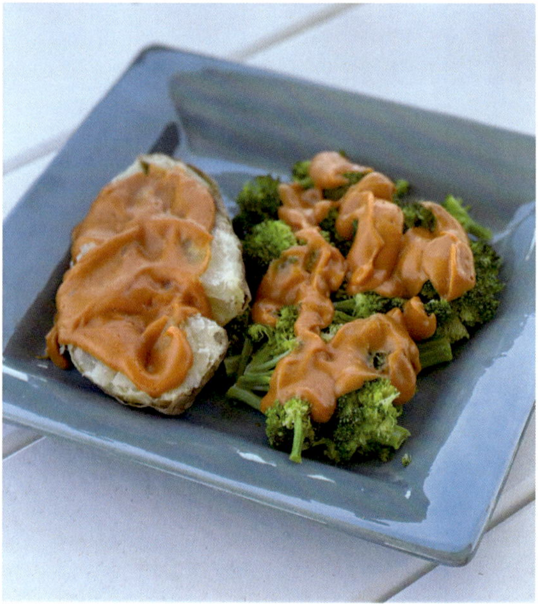

SIMPLE CREAMY DRESSING

This is a light and flavorful salad dressing that can also be used over steamed vegetables or mashed potatoes. The beans make a nice addition of protein and provide a smooth creamy texture.

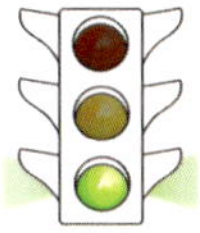

PREP TIME	COOK TIME	YIELD
5 Minutes	N/A	16 oz

INGREDIENTS:

1/2 cup crushed pineapple (in juice)

1/8 cup white wine vinegar

1/4 teaspoon crushed red pepper flakes

1 cup cannellini beans, cooked, drained, and reserve liquid

1/4 cup aquafaba (liquid from beans)

1 tablespoon fresh lemon juice

INSTRUCTIONS:

Place all ingredients in a blender and blend until smooth.

Adjust red pepper flakes or pineapple to your preferred flavor.

Add more aquafaba or water for a thinner consistency.

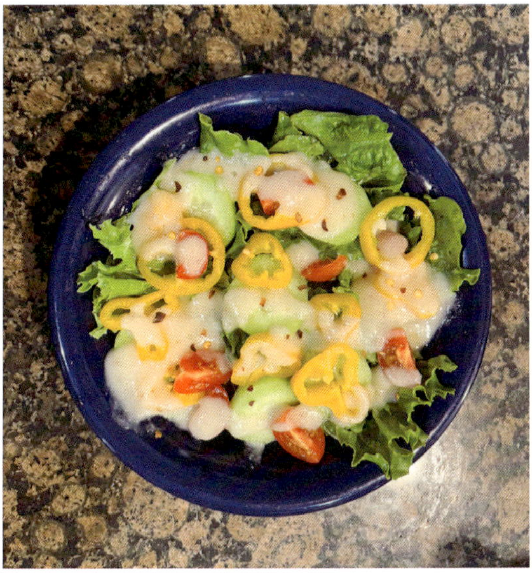

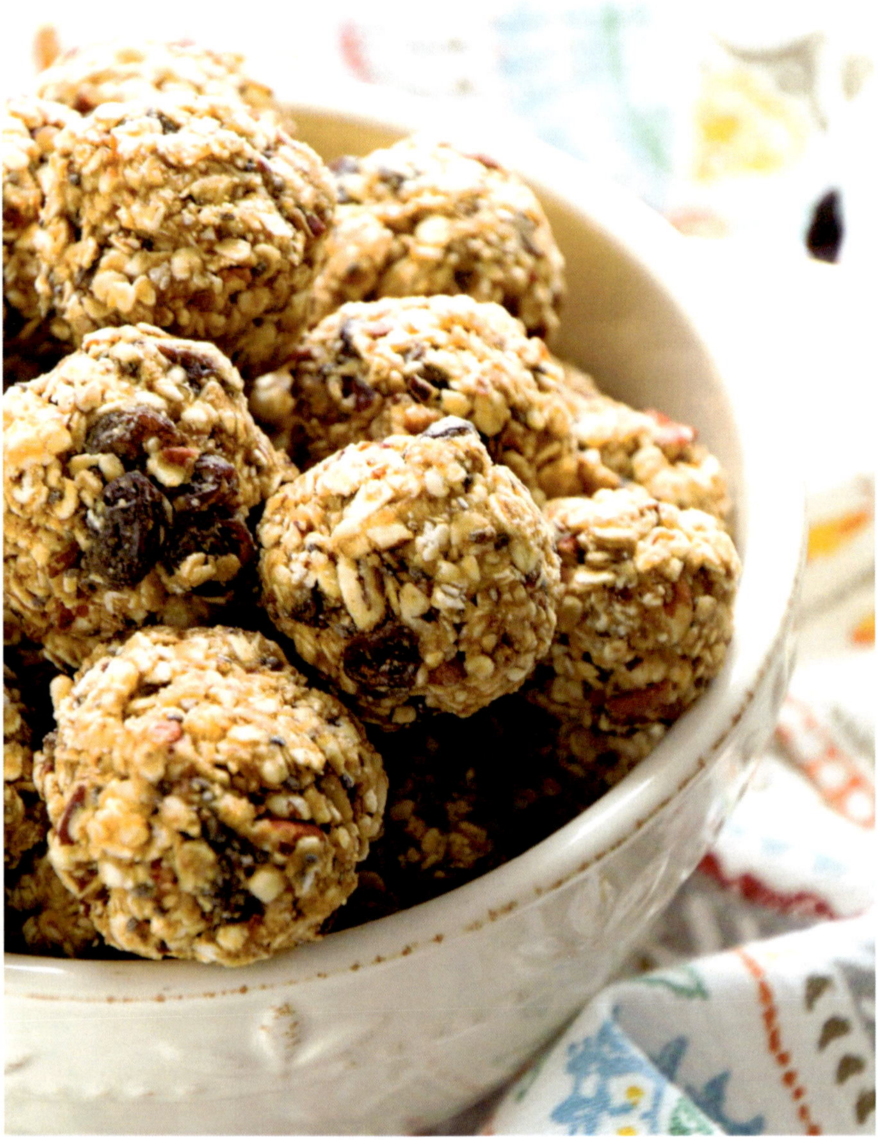

Sweet Treats

THE NOURISHING GREEN SMOOTHIE

This was one of my first green smoothies when I renamed my blog The Nourishing Life. It's kid-tested and mom-approved!

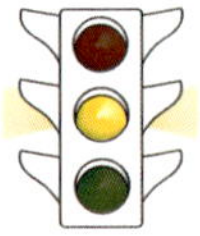

PREP TIME	COOK TIME	YIELD
3 Minutes	N/A	2 8oz. smoothies

INGREDIENTS:

2 cups chopped spinach (frozen)

3/4 cup black beans (really, trust me on this one!)

1 cup unsweetened soy or almond milk

2 bananas (frozen)

1 tablespoon roasted flax seed, ground

1 teaspoon cinnamon

3 dates

INSTRUCTIONS:

Combine all ingredients in high powered blender and blend it until smooth.

Add non-dairy milk slowly, and adjust quantity or add water to desired consistency.

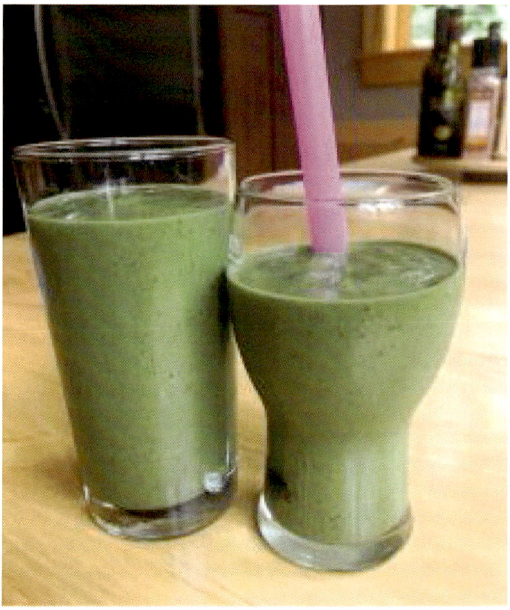

BANANA BREAD SMOOTHIE

This smoothie was inspired by a desire for the delicious sweetness of banana bread, without all the calories. And, because a green smoothie just feels healthier, this one has spinach in it too!

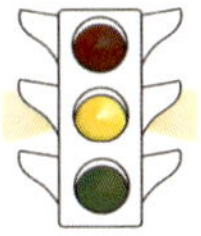

PREP TIME	COOK TIME	YIELD
5 Minutes	N/A	2 8oz. smoothies

INGREDIENTS:

1 1/2 ripe bananas

1/2 cup unsweetened almond milk

1/4 cup raw cashews

2 big handfuls fresh spinach

1 tablespoon hemp seeds

2 dates, pitted

1 teaspoon cinnamon

1/2 teaspoon vanilla

1 1/2 cups ice

INSTRUCTIONS:

Place all ingredients except ice in high speed blender. Blend until smooth and creamy.

Add ice and blend again.

Serve and enjoy immediately.

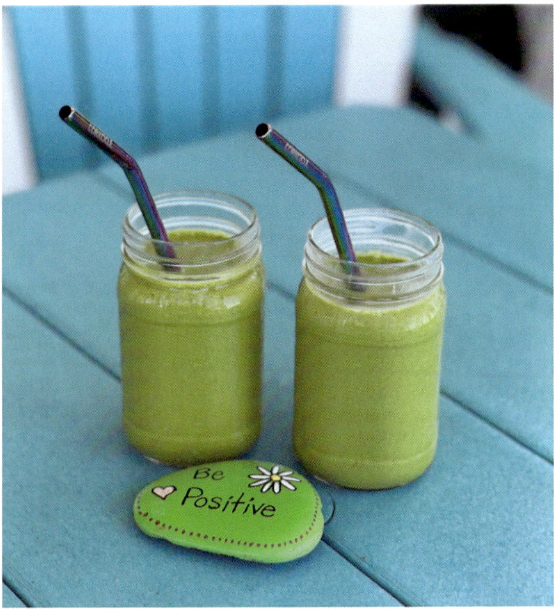

RISE AND SHINE SMOOTHIE

I love a smoothie post-workout, and it's a great option for kids or kids at heart who just can't get enough veggies in any other way. Drink up!

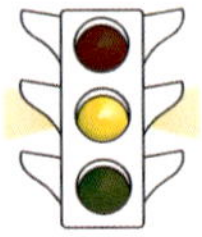

PREP TIME	COOK TIME	YIELD
5 Minutes	N/A	3 8oz. smoothies

INGREDIENTS:

2 cups frozen chopped kale

1 banana, peeled

3/4 cup peaches, frozen (or frozen berries)

1 small orange, peeled

1/4 cup tofu

1/4 cup orange juice

1 cup non-dairy milk

1 teaspoon cinnamon

1 cup ice

1 tablespoon hemp, chia, ground flax seed (optional)

INSTRUCTIONS:

Place all ingredients in high speed blender. Blend on high for 1 minute or until desired consistency.

Serve immediately and enjoy.

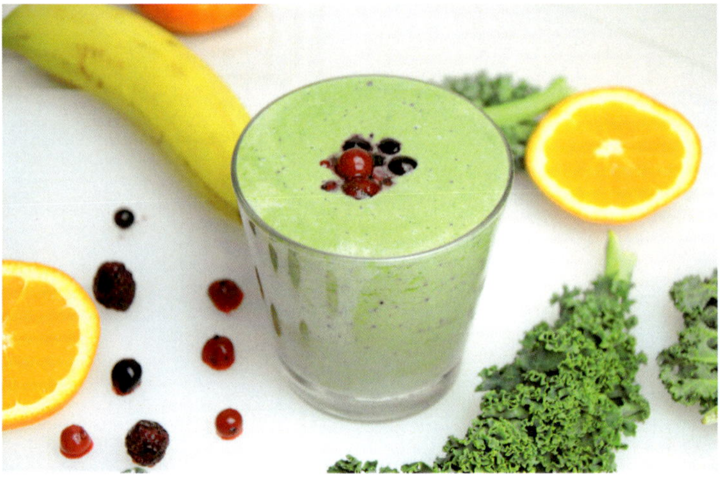

BANANA BREAD OVERNIGHT OATS

Make a batch or two of this oatmeal and you'll have a "home-cooked" breakfast ready to grab and go! No more babysitting oats over the stovetop and reheating a gummy mess the next day. This will easily maintain its texture and delicious flavor!

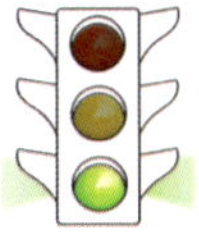

PREP TIME	REFRIGERATE	YIELD
2 Minutes	Overnight	2 8oz. smoothies

INGREDIENTS:

2 cups rolled oats

2 bananas, mashed

2 cups non-dairy milk

2 tablespoons chia seeds or ground flax seeds (optional)

2 teaspoons cinnamon

1/4 teaspoon cardamom

INSTRUCTIONS:

Place all ingredients except ice in high speed blender. Blend until smooth and creamy.

Add ice and blend again.

Serve and enjoy immediately.

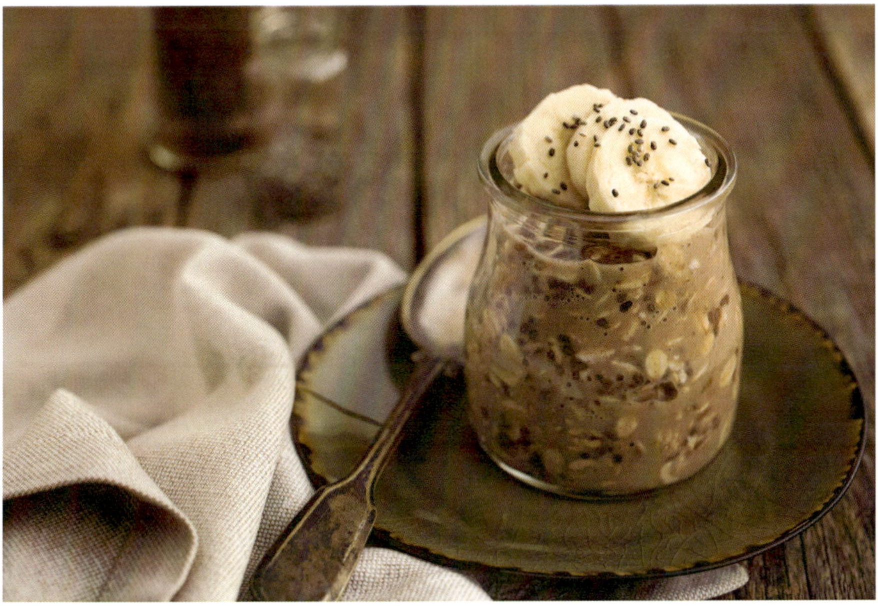

PUMPKIN PIE SMOOTHIE

When you're feeling like pumpkin pie, but you just don't need the calories! This will fill the desire without packing on the pounds.

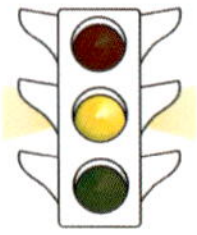

PREP TIME	COOK TIME	YIELD
3 Minutes	N/A	2 oz. smoothies

INGREDIENTS:

1 cup canned pumpkin

2 cups almond milk

1 cup ice cubes

1/2 cup chopped dates

1/2 teaspoon vanilla

1/2 teaspoon cinnamon

pinch nutmeg

INSTRUCTIONS:

Blend all ingredients in high powered blender until smooth.

Drink and enjoy!

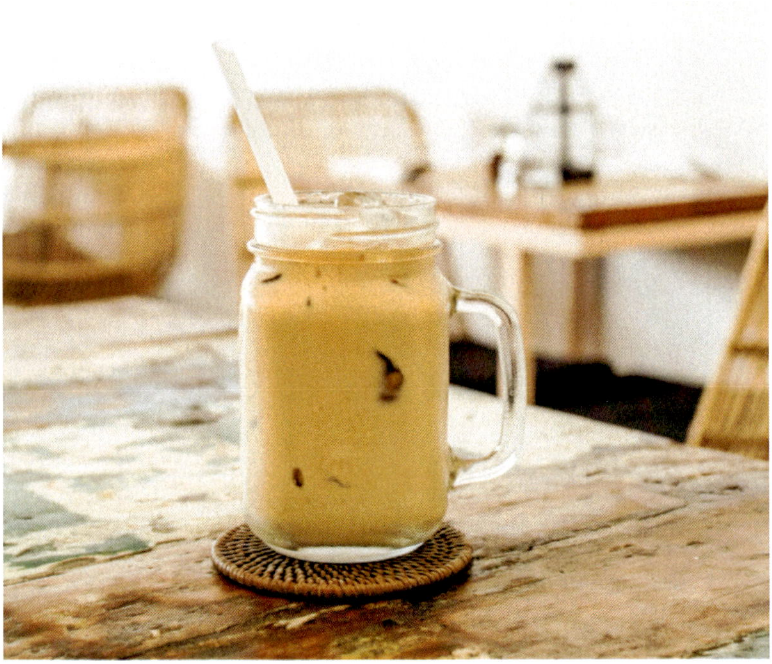

PEACH BERRY COBBLER

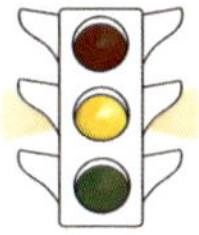

Early one summer I fell into some fresh home-grown peaches. LOTS of them. I ran out of things to make with them, until I developed this recipe. This became breakfast and dessert almost every day until the peach tree was done bearing fruit for the year! It never gets old!

PREP TIME	COOK TIME	YIELD
12 Minutes	25-30 Minutes	4-6 Servings

FILLING INGREDIENTS:

3 cups fresh peaches, sliced

1 cup berries (fresh or frozen, any kind will work!)

1 cup unsweetened applesauce

2 tablespoons ground roasted flax seed (optional)

TOPPING INGREDIENTS:

2 large ripe bananas, mashed

1/4 cup almond milk

2 cups rolled oats

1 tablespoon cinnamon

1 teaspoon cardamom

INSTRUCTIONS:

Preheat oven to 350 degrees.

Combine all filling ingredients directly in a 8×8 or 9×9 baking pan.

In a mixing bowl, combine all topping ingredients.

Put the topping ingredients on top of the filling.

Bake at 350 for 25-30 minutes until topping is starting to brown and fruit is bubbling around the edges.

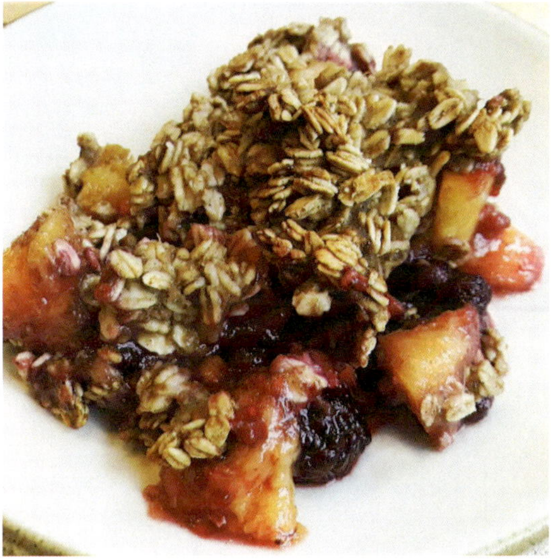

JAPANESE BERRY SURPRISE

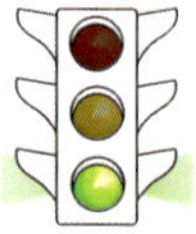

Here it is, the moment you've been waiting for. This is where it gets weird - potatoes for dessert. Hear me out. This is one of the tastiest desserts I've ever served. It's creative, full of flavor, and sweet but not-too-sweet. Oh, and it has to be the healthiest dessert on the planet! A Japanese Sweet Potato topped with antioxidant-rich berries. Sweet, yet satisfying!

PREP TIME	COOK TIME	YIELD
2 Minutes	95 Minutes	As many as your heart desires

INGREDIENTS:

japanese sweet potatoes

frozen berries: blackberries, raspberries, blueberries, or any combination you love

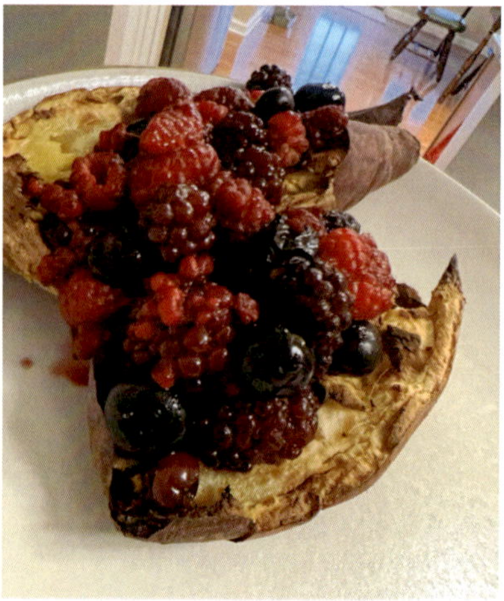

INSTRUCTIONS:

Preheat oven to 375 degrees.

Wash potatoes and arrange on baking tray with non-stick silicone baking mat. Do not prick skins!

Roast for 90 minutes.

Remove from oven.

Without cutting all the way through, slice potatoes lengthwise. Press ends together to open up the middle.

Defrost frozen berries and heat on the stovetop or microwave just to warm.

Spoon warm berries and their juice onto potato and sprinkle with cinnamon.

Note: Save time by roasting a whole tray (or 2) of potatoes at once. Store them in the fridge, standing upright in an open container so they don't get soggy. When you're ready for this dessert or another preparation, you've gotten the time consuming roasting part out of the way! Simply pull one out, reheat in the microwave, and you're done in 5 minutes.

NO-BAKE FUDGE BROWNIES

This recipe was born out of a desire to create a yummy vegan treat for my daughter's school party that wasn't total junk food! You've got to try it to believe it!

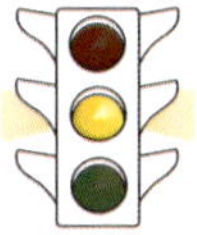

PREP TIME	COOK TIME	YIELD
15 Minutes	30 Minutes	12 Brownies

INGREDIENTS:

1 cup oats, ground

12 medjool dates, pitted

2 cups black beans, rinsed, but save water (aquafaba)

1/2 cup sauerkraut, rinsed & pressed

1/2 cup shredded coconut

1/2 cup carob powder

1 tablespoon vanilla

4-6 tablespoons aquafaba

1/2 cup walnuts, chopped (optional)

1/4 cup dairy-free chocolate chips (optional)

INSTRUCTIONS:

Place all ingredients except walnuts and chocolate chips in food processor.

Process to combine ingredients until smooth, scraping sides as needed.

Add walnuts and chocolate chips if using and pulse a few times.

Spread in 9x13" glass baking dish.

Refrigerate 30 minutes if possible.

Note: For a different twist, add 2 drops peppermint essential oil.

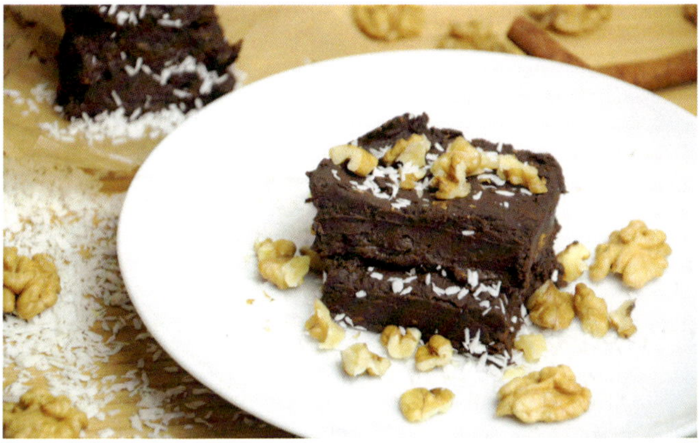

FRESH MINT NICE CREAM

When you're looking for a fresh and cool dessert that wows your guests, tastes delicious, and is more refreshing than sweet, this is the one! You won't even believe how simple it is to prepare.

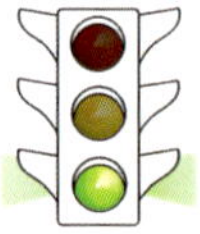

PREP TIME	COOK TIME	YIELD
5 Minutes	N/A	2 Servings

INGREDIENTS:

2 bananas, frozen

1 bunch spinach, stems removed

6-8 mint leaves

1/8 cup plant based milk

4-5 ice cubes

chocolate balsamic vinegar (optional)

INSTRUCTIONS:

Place all ingredients except balsamic vinegar in high speed blender.

Use tamper to press ingredients down into the blade as it begins to mix.

Continue blending until ice cream is green with very few pieces visible.

Add more milk or ice cubes to adjust texture to your preference.

Serve in ice cream bowl.

Drizzle with chocolate balsamic vinegar. Garnish with mint leaves.

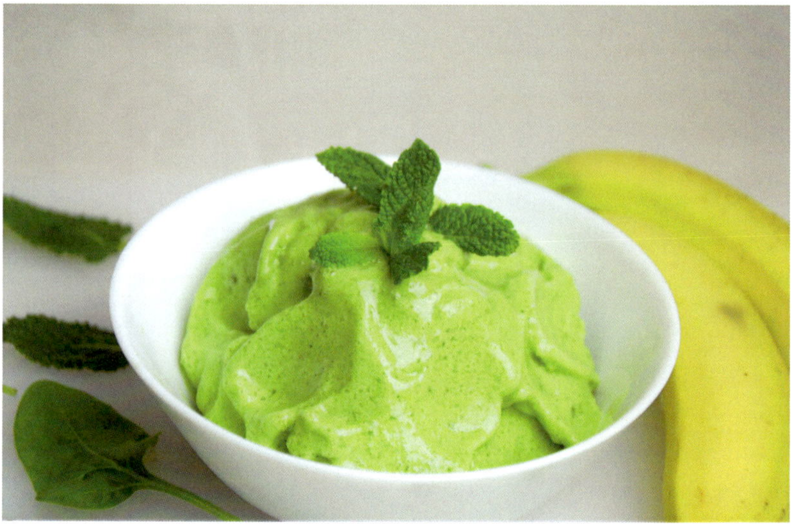

CHOCOLATE CASHEW NICE CREAM

If you're looking for a decadent treat, this is for you. It's also a great one to win kids over to some non-dairy alternatives. You're welcome!

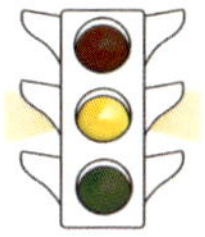

PREP TIME	COOK TIME	YIELD
5 Minutes	N/A	2 Servings

INGREDIENTS:

1/2 cup cashews

2 1/2 frozen bananas

1 tablespoon hemp seed

1/4 cup unsweetened almond milk

2 tablespoons baking cocoa or carob powder

INSTRUCTIONS:

Soak cashews in almond milk in high speed blender and let sit as long as you can stand it (ideally an hour or two, but I know that's not always feasible. It'll work even if you rush it, but it won't be as smooth).

Add bananas and hemp seed and blend until smooth.

Add cocoa powder and blend on low speed until color is consistent.

Note: You certainly can add the cocoa powder along with everything else but I find it just puffs up into a big cloud and doesn't end up quite where it's supposed to be!

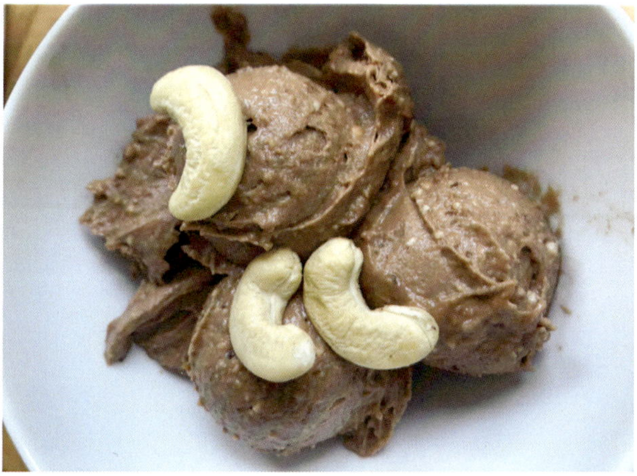

COOKIE DOUGH BALLS

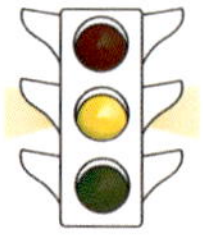

You know how everyone loves to eat cookie dough, but when there are raw eggs it's really not the best idea? And even if the recipe is vegan, you'd feel a little naughty eating cookie dough, right? Well what if you could eat cookie dough that was made with beans and heart-healthy oats? Go ahead and eat your heart out! These taste like oatmeal raisin as the base recipe, or chocolate chip cookie dough with the optional carob chips

PREP TIME	COOK TIME	YIELD
10 Minutes	N/A	2 dozen balls

INGREDIENTS:

2 cups rolled oats

6 pitted medjool dates

1 can cannellini beans, save water when you drain them!

1 teaspoon cinnamon

1/4 teaspoon nutmeg

2 tablespoons aquafaba - the bean water you saved

3 tablespoons unsweetened carob chips, optional

Pictured on Page 56

INSTRUCTIONS:

Place all ingredients except aquafaba in food processor and blend until smooth.

Add the bean water as needed to achieve desired consistency. Dough will start to form a ball on the blade.

Roll into 1 tablespoon balls and serve immediately or store in refrigerator.

Note: If they don't hold together well, add more liquid 1/2 tablespoon at a time until they do.

POWERMINT PATTIES

As with many of my creations, this recipe was inspired by a store-bought product that I had bought a couple times for my daughter, and then instantly regretted it! It was actually the Lara Bar flavor called Mint Chocolate Brownie. It's sweet but not overpowering, and the burst of mint is actually refreshing.

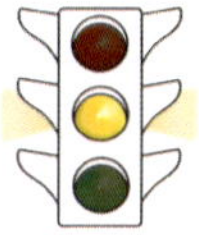

PREP TIME	COOK TIME	YIELD
5 Minutes	N/A	2 Dozen Balls

INGREDIENTS:

1 1/2 cups black beans, (reserve liquid) drained and rinsed

2 cups rolled oats

5 pitted Medjool dates (1/2 cup)

2 tablespoons carob powder

2 drops peppermint essential oil

2-4 tablespoons liquid from beans

INSTRUCTIONS:

Place all the ingredients in a food processor except the liquid from the beans.

Process 2-3 min low speed, scraping sides occasionally.

Process until the mixture begins to form a ball on the blade, adding liquid from the beans. 1 tablespoon at a time as necessary.

Use a scoop to form small balls with your hand and flatten (if desired) to look more like peppermint patties.

Store in the refrigerator.

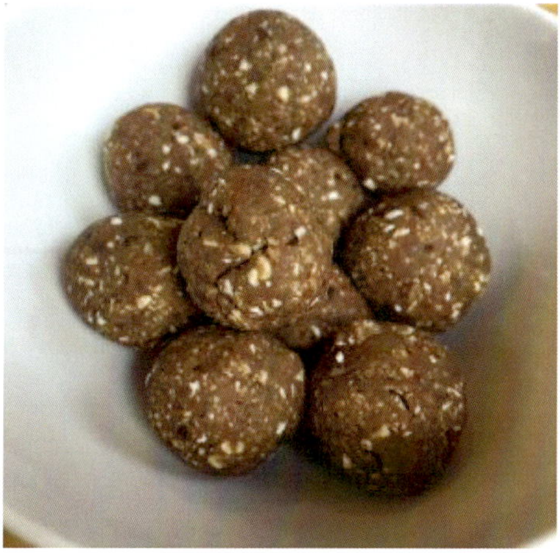

About Christin

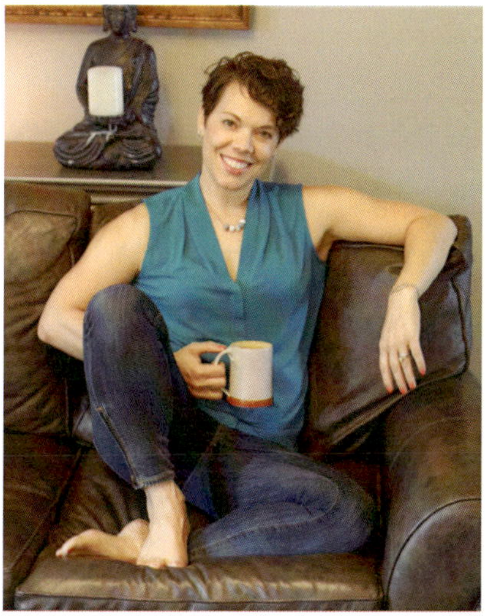

Christin Bummer was diagnosed with hypertension and early insulin resistance at age 32, despite being active and otherwise healthy. It was a massive wake-up call to realize she was walking right down a well-worn path to a family medical history full of heart disease and diabetes. She adopted a whole food plant-based lifestyle, reclaimed her health, lost excess weight, and felt on top of the world! And a few years later she got pregnant and had some difficulties sticking with the plan.

A series of stressful life events pulled her back into old damaging habits, and she found herself really lost, knowing that she wanted to get back on track yet feeling completely unable to do it. Her journey of self-discovery led her to repeatable success, and she's dedicated her life to helping other women overcome similar battles with self-sabotage, insecurities, procrastination, and so much more.

Christin created The Forever Diet online coaching programs now reaching across the globe and she also supports her hometown community with many volunteer endeavors. She is a devoted wife, mom, and cat-mom, and when she's not writing or coaching you'll find her racing up and down the monkey bars with her daughter, hiking in the woods, or daydreaming about their next vacation.